ADVENTURE
READY

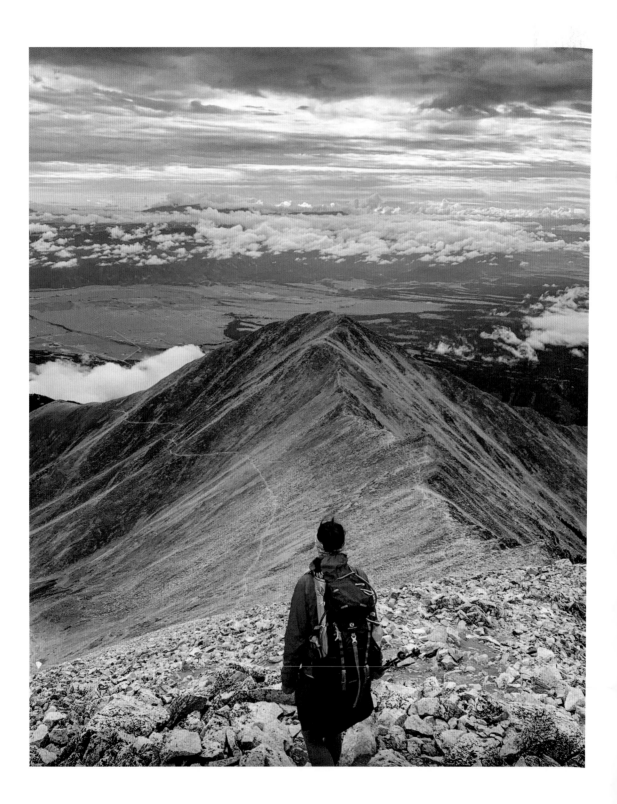

ADVENTURE READY

A HIKER'S GUIDE TO PLANNING, TRAINING & RESILIENCY

KATIE GERBER & HEATHER ANDERSON

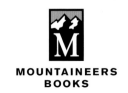

MOUNTAINEERS BOOKS

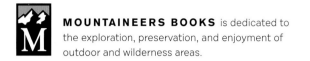

MOUNTAINEERS BOOKS is dedicated to the exploration, preservation, and enjoyment of outdoor and wilderness areas.

1001 SW Klickitat Way, Suite 201, Seattle, WA 98134
800-553-4453, mountaineersbooks. org

Printed in China
Distributed in the United Kingdom by Cordee, www.cordee.co.uk
First edition, 2022

Copyeditor: Erin Cusick
Design and layout: Kate Basart/Union Pageworks
All photographs by the authors unless credited otherwise
Cover photograph: Left: *The Sierra Buttes from Deer Lake* (photo by Philip Kramer); Right: *Hiker on the Los Angeles Aqueduct section of the Pacific Crest Trail* (photo by Tommy Corey)
Frontispiece: *Adventure awaits!*

Library of Congress Cataloging-in-Publication data is on file for this title at https://lccn.loc.gov/2021039974. The ebook record is available at https://lccn.loc.gov/2021039975.

Mountaineers Books titles may be purchased for corporate, educational, or other promotional sales, and our authors are available for a wide range of events. For information on special discounts or booking an author, contact our customer service at 800-553-4453 or mbooks@ mountaineersbooks.org.

Printed on FSC®-certified materials

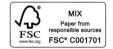

MIX
Paper from
responsible sources
FSC® C001701

ISBN (paperback): 978-1-68051-544-2
ISBN (ebook): 978-1-68051-545-9

An independent nonprofit publisher since 1960

CONTENTS

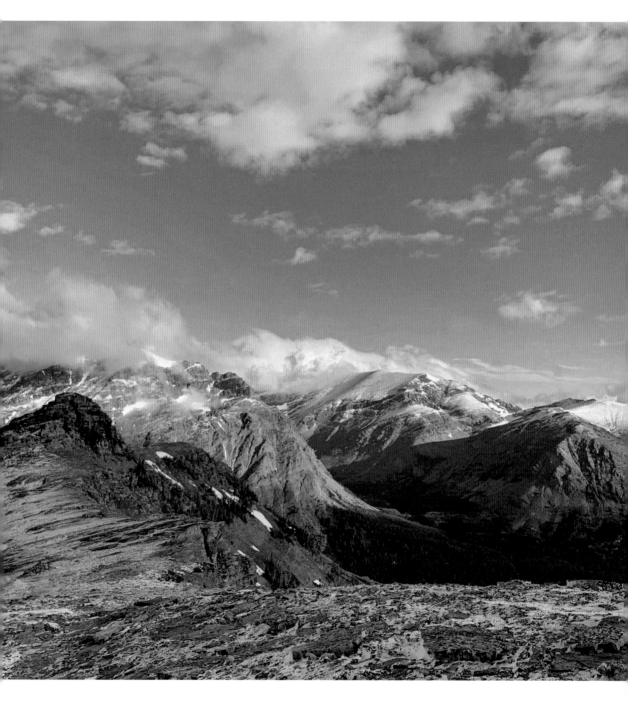

Parting clouds after an early morning snow shower on the Continental Divide Trail in Glacier National Park

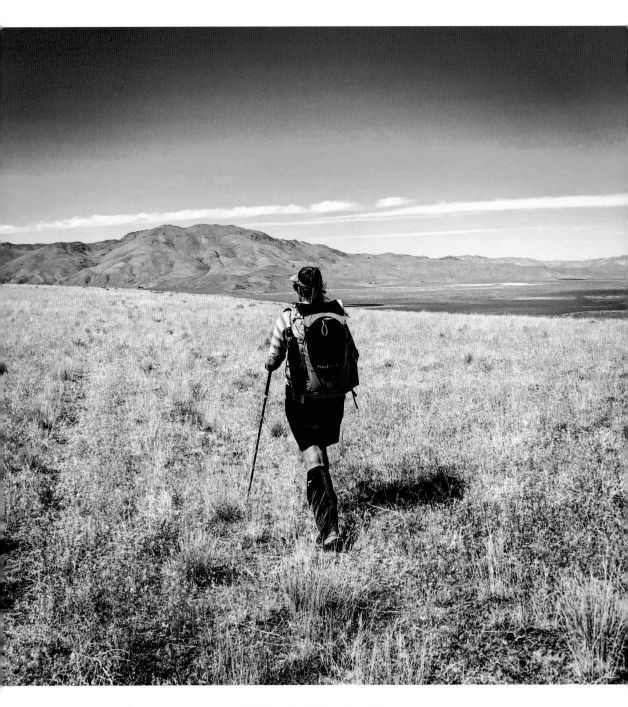

Cross-country hiking on the Oregon Desert Trail (Photo by Whitney LaRuffa)

INTRODUCTION: TIME TO GET ADVENTURE READY!

Even after nearly two decades, I (Katie) can vividly recall the excitement I felt the first night I slept in the backcountry. I had never experienced such contentment as I did at the end of a day spent walking through the woods, moving my body as humans are meant to, the sun soaking into my skin, fresh air in my lungs, with nature's symphony filling my ears. Unplugging from the incessant onslaught of news, to-do lists, and ever present distractions felt somehow forbidden—and incredibly intoxicating. I didn't grow up backpacking, and the knowledge and skills I now have were learned the hard way. However, with each trip, I deepened my understanding of the natural world and the planning, gear, navigation, training, and safety measures required to immerse myself in it. I found myself exploring the wilderness with increasing confidence. The more comfortable I became in the backcountry, the more present I could be, taking in the fullness of my time spent in nature. While there's no substitute for direct experience, my hope is that the concepts in this book enable you to embark on your next adventure with a greater sense of preparedness, so that you can have your own unique experience in the outdoors.

Like Katie, I (Heather) did not grow up hiking, and when I began backpacking in the early 2000s, there weren't a ton of resources, at least when it came to long-distance backpacking, so I learned through trial and error. This learning process was a sometimes painful experience that resulted in lost toenails, pack bruising, blisters, and malnutrition. Yet I loved the experience of spending days, weeks, and months in nature with all I needed in my backpack, so I kept coming back. With each trip I learned more about gear, nutrition, my physical abilities, and how to be safe and content in the woods. The path from neophyte to seasoned backpacker was steep, but today I step onto the trail the same way I walk into my living room—with ease and comfort. My journey was not unique, and I hope that, with the help of this book, your learning curve will be a bit more gently graded.

Adventure Ready: A Hiker's Guide to Planning, Training & Resiliency is the outgrowth of our Adventure Ready online courses which include a holistic hiker course, Adventure Ready, that is a step-by-step guide to creating resilient health before any adventure, as well as Backpacker Academy, which teaches the outdoor skills necessary to safely and confidently explore the backcountry. This book covers similar topics, and you can use it on its own or in conjunction with the more immersive online courses.

The mission behind Adventure Ready is to empower others by synthesizing our own experiences as hikers, runners, and outdoor adventurers with our unique expertise in nutrition and personal training. This guidebook provides a step-by-step approach to learning the basics of gear selection, navigation, and trip planning, as well as nutritional and physical preparation. On top of that, *Adventure Ready* prepares you for the emotional and mental challenges of spending several weeks or months in the backcountry.

We believe that longer journeys in nature can be life-changing and a gateway to experiencing more of your true self. Together, we hope that this book gives you the tools to become adventure ready!

KATIE'S STORY

On a drizzly morning in March 2009, I stood under the stone archway at Amicalola Falls State Park, my body propping up the weight of a 55-pound pack full of borrowed gear. I was joining a college friend for the beginning of his Appalachian Trail (AT) thru-hike. At that point in my life, I had been on exactly one overnight backpacking trip ever, and until a few months prior, was unaware of the existence of the AT and the world of long-distance hiking. I had no idea what would come of this adventure, but I was excited.

I hiked 600 miles of the AT that year before a family emergency pulled me back home. But in those six weeks, the trajectory of my life shifted. During those weeks of extended time in nature, I found a connection with myself and the surrounding world that I didn't know I'd been missing. I felt like I was where I belonged for the first time in a long time, and I fell in love with the experience and culture of thru-hiking. I also discovered that there were more trails like the AT, trails covering thousands of miles at a stretch, all over the world. A seed was planted, and I had a strong sense that long-distance hiking would become an integral part of my life.

It took five years for me to find my way back to a long trail—this time the Pacific Crest Trail (PCT)—through the serendipitous ways of the universe. I was working as a baker near Asheville, North Carolina, at the time, staying busy with daily routine and believing that I was content enough. But on my evening and weekend runs through the wooded trails of the Appalachians, I could hear my inner voice calling for greater freedom and adventure.

On Memorial Day of 2013, I was bitten by a rattlesnake while out on a run. I was bedridden for three weeks with my swollen black-and-blue

A NOTE ABOUT SAFETY

Please use common sense. This book is not intended as a substitute for professional medical advice, physical training, careful planning, and/or your own good judgment. It is incumbent upon any user of this guide to assess his or her own skills, experience, fitness, and equipment. Readers will recognize the inherent dangers found in wilderness settings and when hiking, backpacking, or pursuing other outdoor adventures, and assume responsibility for their own actions and safety. Changing or unfavorable conditions in weather, waterways, roads, trails, etc. cannot be anticipated by the authors or publisher but should be considered by any outdoor participants, as routes may become dangerous or unstable due to such altered conditions. Likewise, be aware of any changes in public jurisdiction, and do not access private property without permission.

The authors have made every effort to ensure the accuracy of the information provided in this book; however, nutrition and exercise research is constantly evolving, so changes in information, facts, and/or recommendations described herein may also have changed. Ultimately, this book contains the personal opinions and experiences of the authors shared for educational and inspirational purposes only. The publisher and authors are expressly not responsible for any adverse consequences resulting directly or indirectly from information contained in this book.

—Mountaineers Books

leg propped up on pillows. During that time, a friend dropped a book off for me: *Called Again* by Jennifer Pharr Davis. The author had given my friend the book earlier that day during a chance encounter at the bakery where we both worked. Sometimes certain books, stories, or people enter your life at just the right moment and pour fuel onto a small fire that was already burning within you. I devoured the book in forty-eight hours, my love of long-distance hiking reignited. As I turned the final page, I committed to being on another long-distance trail as soon as possible and to never again going so many years without satisfying that thirst for extended time in the outdoors.

The following year, I thru-hiked the PCT and it was as fulfilling as I'd hoped it would be, but I returned home feeling extremely fatigued. According to doctors, I was fine. But I knew I was not. My deepest longing at the time was to get my body ready for adventure again, so I began reading medical journals, scientific articles, and books by doctors and other experts to find possible causes for my symptoms. I ordered my own labs online and began to experiment with different protocols. As part of my learning, I apprenticed with a functional medicine practitioner, and completed a nutrition certification as well as an herbal medicine certification. My health began to improve, and I was slowly able to return to the active outdoor life that I love.

Since then, I've been on many amazing adventures, including thru-hikes of the Colorado Trail, Continental Divide Trail (CDT), Oregon Desert Trail, and Wind River High Route. With each trail, I have expanded my skill set and learned more about preparing for backcountry adventures and staying safe and healthy in the process.

Once I made progress in my own health journey, I wanted to support others for whom health challenges were an obstacle to actualizing their outdoor adventure dreams. Extended excursions in nature had become a central part of my life, and I knew the frustration of not having

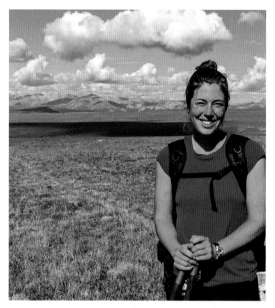

Katie Gerber in her element on Snow Mesa, Colorado

the health to do the thing I loved—the thing that made me feel like myself. I knew there must be others who felt similarly. The idea for the first Adventure Ready course originated with those post-PCT health challenges and my desire to regain vitality so that I could get back to hiking, running, and exploring the wild again. I resolved to help others achieve resilient health and enjoy the gift of extended time in the outdoors.

In working toward that vision, I started an online business coaching clients one-on-one in nutrition and holistic health, and I shared what I'd learned through my blog. Through client and reader feedback, I realized that the principles that had helped me become adventure ready again weren't only useful to someone dealing with a chronic health condition: they were just as impactful for anyone wanting to create optimal health before and during a big adventure.

In an effort to reach more people than was possible in a one-to-one setting, I decided the best approach was to package these ideas in an online course. I had an idea for what I wanted it to be and I created an outline, but I delayed taking further action because I knew there needed to be a physical training component to the course if it were to truly be a holistic physical preparation guide for backpackers. Though I'd been an athlete my whole life, I had no formal training in the subject.

All of this was percolating at the time I hiked the Oregon Desert Trail. I was sharing the course idea with my hiking partner one day as we walked through miles of sagebrush on an endless dirt road. "Do you know Heather Anderson?" he asked. I didn't. "She's a thru-hiker and personal trainer. You two would be the perfect team." A few weeks later, after the end of our hike, he put me in touch with Heather. I proposed the course idea and the prospect of a collaboration—and happily, she said yes!

That original course was the beginning of a fruitful friendship and partnership. I never imagined the Adventure Ready concept would grow into a family of courses, an online community, and now a book. It's an honor and a gift to have the opportunity to continue to share these ideas with you.

My hope is that this book will empower you on your backcountry adventures and help you avoid many of the mistakes that I made. In addition to a new skill set, long-distance hiking has given me a greater sense of self-reliance and a deeper knowledge of who I am and what I'm truly capable of. May your adventures be similarly fruitful.

Through my holistic health and nutrition coaching practice, I now have the pleasure and honor of helping others to create optimal health and prepare for their own backcountry adventures. The Adventure Ready platform has now expanded beyond physical preparation and nutrition to include courses on backcountry skills, such as navigation and safety. This how-to guide, my first book, is a natural complement to the more immersive online curriculum.

When I'm not working with clients through private health and nutrition coaching, online courses, and as a backpacking guide, I'm hiking, running, backpacking, or skiing in the mountains surrounding my home in Colorado.

HEATHER'S STORY

In May of 2003, I set out on the AT from Springer Mountain in Georgia, planning to walk more than 2000 miles to Mount Katahdin in Maine. At that time, I had done only a few day-hiking trips and a couple of overnights. I was wearing a 40-pound pack full of everything I didn't need . . . and nothing I did! But I did have plenty of curiosity and desire to go on a grand adventure.

Despite the fact that I was underprepared, I made it to the end of that hike four months later. It was the most formative experience of my life. Along that trail I learned many of the skills needed to be a successful long-distance hiker. I also learned about the worldviews and lifestyles of a wide array of fellow hikers. It was like traveling the world without leaving my home country. While I hiked, I also learned something else vitally important: there were other long-distance hiking trails. I made it my life's goal to hike as many of them as I could, regardless of whether it meant giving up what I'd considered "normal" life goals prior to that moment.

This commitment to hiking for life is what led me to return to complete the AT twice more, as well as the PCT and CDT each three times (and counting!). Completing this "Triple Crown" of backpacking three times—with one of those completions occurring all in one calendar year—made me the first woman to achieve either of these goals. Along the way I set fastest known times (FKTs) on several different trails, notably the PCT and AT, and I was named the Fastest Known Time of the Year Athlete by Ultimate Direction in 2016. In 2019, I was also selected as a National Geographic Adventurer of the Year for my Calendar-Year Triple Crown.

But the thing about the accolades is that they attempt to label something that cannot be labeled. Long-distance backpacking for me has always been both an adventure and a homecoming. Spending months on end in nature can clear your mind, help you gain perspective, and teach you self-reliance that you cannot learn elsewhere. With this book, I hope to provide tools for more people to find adventure and truth in nature.

My route to sharing my backcountry knowledge did not start with this guide. After setting some FKTs, I knew I wanted to have a career that focused on sharing what I'd learned. In 2015, I became a personal trainer and began coaching clients on the physical preparation for their long-distance treks. It was incredibly fulfilling. However, I could reach only so many people, and with frequent long-distance hikes on my

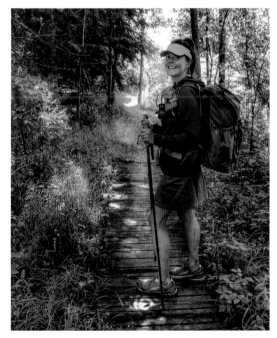

Heather Anderson enjoying the trail

own itinerary, I realized that I no longer had time to coach. When Katie reached out to me about collaborating on a holistic training course for long-distance hikers, I knew it was the opportunity I'd been waiting for, and Adventure Ready was born. It's amazing to see how far those ideas have gone, how they've grown—culminating not only in popular online courses but also this book.

I have been thrilled to contribute my training knowledge to a course that could help more people than I'd ever be able to coach individually, and as the Adventure Ready family of courses has continued to grow, I have been able to share more than just my knowledge about performance but also the wisdom of experience.

Distilling the essence of those courses into book format has been another way to make sure it reaches even more people. This book can work in tandem with the courses, which go more in depth on several topics, and yet each stands alone in its completeness. Through these varied channels I have the opportunity to present you with the lessons I've learned over nearly two decades of long-distance-hiking experiences.

My hiking did not stop with the Triple Crown of backpacking. In fact, hiking those three trails for the first time instilled in me the lifelong love of wild travel through the mountains, and I have continued to hike, backpack, mountaineer, and trail run through the wild spaces of the United States and multiple other countries. In 2020, I finished my fifteenth thru-hike by completing a southbound traverse of the 300-mile-long Benton MacKaye Trail—finishing at its southern terminus on Springer Mountain, seventeen years after starting my first AT adventure there.

When I am not out hiking, running, or ascending mountains, I am a professional speaker and writer, the author of two memoirs: *Thirst: 2600 Miles to Home* (chronicling my PCT record) and *Mud, Rocks, Blazes: Letting Go on the Appalachian Trail* (2021) about my 2015 AT record. *Adventure Ready* is my first guidebook.

HOW TO USE THIS BOOK

This guide is designed to prepare beginner to intermediate backpackers and aspiring thru-hikers for success while saving them time, money, and mistakes. If you're an experienced backpacker, this book will help you learn to apply your skills to long-distance trips. If you're new to backpacking, use this book as a reference as you gain skills and build toward longer backpacking trips.

Backpacking—especially longer trips of weeks or months—is a great way to get exercise and fresh air; it's also an opportunity to reconnect with ourselves and the natural world. Spending long periods of time in nature can reset our stress levels and circadian rhythms, allowing us to feel rejuvenated—even after lugging a backpack over rough terrain!

This comprehensive guide provides the resources you need to prepare for your first long-distance trek—or help you with the things that didn't go so well on a previous one. We cover basic topics such as gear and navigation and also delve into aspects that most guides don't spend much time on, such as nutrition and the mental aspects of long-distance backpacking. Though the chapters of this book are divided with each of us writing about areas in which we have more expertise, we have also included Adventure Tips in each chapter that offer insight on the topic from the other author. No two people are exactly alike, and no two hikers will hike the same hike. We aim to offer different perspectives to many topics throughout the book.

The first two chapters discuss the basics of planning your trip and choosing your gear. Chapter 1 offers a simple, effective framework to help you plan any trip, regardless of distance, location, or season. We cover the key factors to consider to help you define your trip parameters,

research likely conditions, create an itinerary, and prepare for a safe and successful trip. Chapter 2 discusses timeless principles for how to evaluate, select, and test gear so that you can find the right item for *you*. Primary gear items, including packs, shelters, sleep systems, and food preparation, are covered in detail. Sample summer gear lists from each of us are provided for reference.

Chapters 3 and 4 expand on the topics of safety, navigation, and route preparedness. We focus on preparation and mitigation while recognizing the inherent risks of backcountry travel. Learn how to assess various risk factors for your chosen route and learn tools to prepare and mitigate risks as well as the basics of navigation. See Worksheets & Checklists at the back of the book to create your own assessments and beta packets.

Chapters 5 and 6 dive deep into nutrition and nourishing your body before, during, and after the physically demanding effort of a long backpacking trip. Chapter 5 focuses on lifestyle strategies, including gut health, sleep optimization, and stress management, that allow you to create resilient health before stepping foot on trail. Supplementation is covered as well. In chapter 6, you'll learn how to dial in your nutrition at home so you begin your journey fully nourished. Then we outline the key principles of performance nutrition and how to eat for optimal energy, faster recovery, and pack-weight efficiency. Ultralight backcountry meal planning is also covered.

Chapter 7 discusses preparing the physical body for the rigors of the trail. We review the main body systems that benefit from preparatory work and offer some sample exercises and schedules. Maintenance on the trail is also discussed.

Chapters 8 and 9 focus on the mental aspects of long-distance backpacking. The

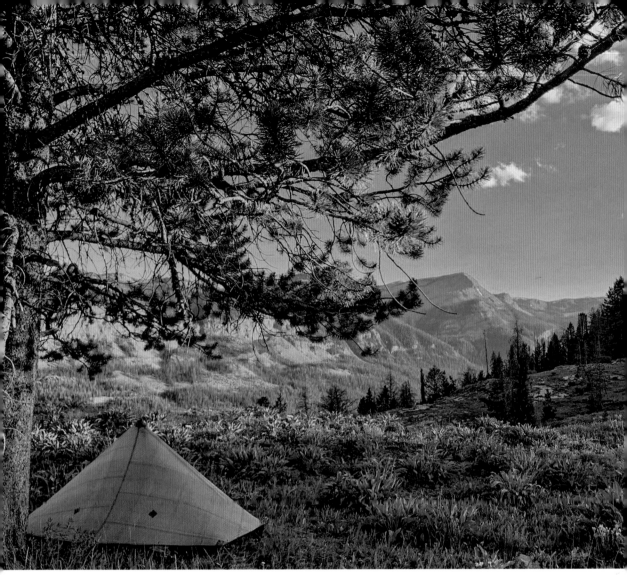

Idyllic campsite on the Continental Divide Trail in Wyoming

mental strain of spending many weeks or months in the backcountry is often underestimated, as is the mental adjustment after the trip ends. These chapters provide tools to prepare yourself mentally for the transition from trail to back home. In both cases, knowing what to expect can be tremendously helpful. A buffet of techniques and strategies is offered for mental preparation (chapter 8) and reintegration (chapter 9), so that you can find what works best.

Finally, we have included a collection of Additional Resources for you to use as you continue to expand your backcountry skill set. Selected Sources provides a list of research references.

Not every reader will need every topic, so feel free to pick and choose which chapters apply more to your situation. There is something for everyone in this comprehensive, holistic guide.

1

PLANNING YOUR BACKPACKING TRIP: AN OVERVIEW

BY *Katie*

When I became interested in going on multi-night trips in the backcountry, I quickly learned that planning a backpacking trip is a skill: one that's important to develop if you intend to spend significant time exploring the outdoors. My first backpacking trip was in college as part of a class, and the instructor did all the planning. When I attempted to plan my second-ever multi-night backpacking trip, on the Appalachian National Scenic Trail (AT), I used the knowledge I had gained from that college backpacking course—a very outdated approach as I came to learn—combined with what my hiking partner shared with me based on his research, and I hoped for the best. There were far fewer online resources back then, and I had zero connections to the long-distance hiking world—a world I didn't even know existed. In fact, I had never even heard of the AT when my friend had posed the idea to me five months earlier. I knew only that I needed an escape from my life at the time, I loved the outdoors, and it sounded like a grand adventure. And though the adventure *was* grand, my oversights ended up costing me money, time, and enjoyment.

Since those early days, I've learned a lot about the importance of trip planning and how to do it effectively and efficiently. Now, not only do I love the planning phase because it vastly increases my safety, happiness, and odds of success but it also builds anticipation for the adventure to come!

This chapter covers a straightforward process for planning a multi-week backpacking trip from start to finish—a resource we wish we had had when we got started. We focus primarily on

planning a longer excursion, such as a thru-hike, but there are also tips sprinkled throughout for shorter trips. Following a framework can prevent you from feeling overwhelmed and makes the trip-planning process easier each time. This method involves defining your trip parameters, evaluating likely conditions, creating an itinerary, selecting gear, planning your resupply, understanding backcountry safety, and preparing yourself physically and mentally.

For multi-week to multi-month excursions, your trip planning might begin more than a year out from your projected start date. The amount of time needed to plan will be different for everyone and depends on factors such as your experience, trip complexity, trip duration, destination, and your familiarity with the area. In general, the less experienced you are and

EVALUATE POTENTIAL PRE-TRIP TASKS

Consider the following tasks to help you determine how much planning time you'll need. Not every item on this list will apply to every trip.

- Define trip parameters
- Create a budget and determine how long it will take you to save
- Coordinate plans with hiking partner(s)
- Connect with the hiking community for support
- Research trip conditions
- Order and print maps and guidebooks
- Create a general itinerary
- Book transportation and pre-trip lodging
- Acquire permits and visas
- Research and acquire gear
- Take shakeout hikes and test gear
- Determine a resupply strategy
- Purchase food and prepare resupply boxes
- Create a backcountry safety plan

- Acquire and familiarize yourself with your navigational tools
- Prepare physically
- Prepare mentally and emotionally
- Take courses in wilderness first aid, navigation, snow safety, etc.
- Plan your exit strategy from work
- Identify and arrange tasks to be completed at home before your departure, such as finding someone to care for your pets, plants, or your house; moving your belongings; forwarding or holding mail; putting bills on auto-pay; arranging health insurance, and so on
- Do a final check (see later in this chapter) and get excited!

the greater the complexity and duration of the trip, the more preparation time you will need. For example, a five-month thru-hike of the Pacific Crest National Scenic Trail (PCT) may require a year of planning for someone new to long-distance hiking, whereas a more experienced backpacker may need only two months to plan. The more experience you gain, the easier the planning becomes.

No matter how much experience you have, there is a lot to take care of before a long hike. Always give yourself plenty of time to properly plan. It saves you time overall, money, and hassle once you're out on the trail!

DEFINING TRIP PARAMETERS

Begin by defining the basic parameters of your trip: Where do you want to go? When and with whom? For each of these questions, gather information to make decisions that suit your preferences and allow you to mitigate risk: research potential routes, evaluate the climate and terrain, consider any time constraints you may have, and reflect on whether you prefer to hike solo or with a partner or group.

Where: Choosing Your Route

Whether you already have a specific route in mind or you're still narrowing your options, you can solidify your decision by evaluating factors such as weather and climate, geographic features, skills required, and your preferences regarding social interaction with other hikers.

Climate, Seasons, and Weather

Understanding the climate and seasonal patterns of an area will help you decide when and where it's most appropriate to backpack to experience more favorable conditions. *Climate* refers to the typical weather in a location, generally averaged over a period of thirty years. For example, the desert is hot and dry; mountains tend to be cool and wet. *Seasons* are marked by particular

weather patterns and daylight hours. Even if your travel dates aren't flexible and you have a set window of time available, evaluating climate and season data enables you to choose a route in a region where the conditions will be suitable for backpacking during your chosen time.

If you want to hike the Sierra High Route, for example, and don't have any scheduling restrictions, you will probably want to plan your trip for August, when you're most likely to be there after the snow melts and before it falls again. Alternatively, if you have only the month of March available, your options of viable routes for that time of year will narrow. In that case, you might choose the Grand Enchantment Trail or the Arizona Trail: each is a lower latitude desert hike with more tolerable temperatures and more abundant water in late winter through early spring.

Weather refers to the state of the atmosphere at a place and time with regard to heat, dryness, sunshine, wind, rain, and so forth. It varies by the day—even by the hour. Climate and seasons give you a broader picture of expected conditions while the weather gives you specifics. In the context of planning, weather is more relevant on shorter trips, where you may decide whether or not to go based on the forecast. On a longer trip, it's helpful to check the weather before each leg of your trip as it can help you determine what gear to carry or even if you want to leave town as planned. There are many resources to find current weather conditions. A particularly excellent option in the United States is the National Oceanic and Atmospheric Administration (NOAA; see Additional Resources). Rather than entering the zip code of the nearest town, use the point-and-click map on their website to pinpoint weather at the trailhead, peaks, and points along your route. The weather in the mountains can be much different from the weather in a nearby valley or town.

Gather climate, season, and weather data into a document and cite the source so you can easily access updated information as you continue planning. Take into account average temperatures, record high/low temperatures, average precipitation, record high/low precipitation, precipitation frequency, humidity, wind, and any other seasonal weather patterns (e.g., monsoon season or snowmelt). Consider how these factors will change along your route based on elevation (adjust 3 to 5 degrees for every 1000 vertical feet). You can also use this data to evaluate water accessibility and river crossings so you can plan accordingly.

Geographic Features

What types of features do you want to experience? Mountains, lakes, or waterfalls? High, dry ponderosas, or thick, mossy old growth? For many thru-hikes, such as the AT or PCT, the route is already established and traverses through a range of ecosystems and geographic features. In other instances, you might create your own route or choose one that passes through a specific landscape, such as the desert or high alpine. Keep in mind that certain ecosystems come with specific challenges, such as water availability and sun exposure in the desert, or vertical exposure, unstable terrain like scree fields, and snow-covered passes on high routes.

Requisite Skill Set

Certain routes require unique skill sets, such as technical climbing or off-trail navigation, and the season in which you plan to travel also influences the skills you may need to stay safe. Hiking through an area too early or late in a season increases your risk level and requires specific skills: if you are still on the PCT when winter snowfalls begin, for example, you'll need advanced skills in snow travel and avalanche awareness to safely traverse mountain passes, whereas a summer hike on the same trail is far less risky and is accessible to most individuals. Do your research and choose a route that is within your ability and experience level.

Social Experience

Reflect on how much social interaction or solitude you're seeking. Do you want to go days without seeing another person, or do you want to see other hikers frequently on trail? Knowing your preference can help you determine which route to hike as well as in which direction and during what season. The AT and PCT, for instance, are very social trails, especially if you hike them northbound during the "standard" thru-hiking season of April to September. However, it's quite possible to go days without seeing another person on more remote routes. On the Oregon Desert Trail, I didn't see another hiker apart from my hiking partners for an entire month.

When: Choosing Your Trip Dates

Consider any personal constraints you have, such as school, work, family vacations, or other commitments. These events may affect your start date directly or indirectly. For example, if

WEATHER WINDOWS ON THE TRIPLE CROWN TRAILS				
	NORTHBOUND START	**NORTHBOUND FINISH**	**SOUTHBOUND START**	**SOUTHBOUND FINISH**
APPALACHIAN TRAIL	Mid-March to early May	By mid-October	Early June to mid-July	By mid-November
CONTINENTAL DIVIDE TRAIL	Mid-April to early May	By early October	Mid-June to mid-July	By mid-November
PACIFIC CREST TRAIL	Mid-April to early May	By early October	Mid-June to mid-July	By mid-November

MAKING YOUR DREAM HIKE HAPPEN

Don't be discouraged if you find you have obligations that seem like they may prevent you from hiking your dream route. The options for planning are endless if you're willing to get creative. There are many ways to hike a long-distance trail: You can hike end to end, as in a traditional thru-hike. There's the option to flip-flop hike, where you skip around and hike sections of the trail, piecing it together. And if you don't have the time or interest in hiking the whole route in one season, you may decide to section hike over multiple years. There are pros and cons to each option. Most importantly, it's about finding what works best for you.

you have an internship that lasts until late June, it may not be advisable to start a northbound PCT thru-hike that late in the season; alternatively, if you need to finish before a certain date, such as the start of school in mid-September, you need to be sure you start on a date that allows you to complete the route before then. These types of dates are generally nonnegotiable, so factor them in first as you select your start date.

On long hikes, it's unnecessary to set an exact end date unless you have a personal obligation. It is important, however, to set an approximate end date so that you can plan daily mileage goals and map out an itinerary. In most instances, your ideal end date will be determined by your weather window. On shorter hikes, choose an end date based on daily mileage predictions and the length of your route. It's important to be more accurate with your dates on shorter hikes so that you can arrange transportation and give clear instructions to your emergency contact for when you'll return.

Weather Window

Another factor that affects your start date is the "weather window" for your chosen route. Review season and climate data for your destination to determine the best time to backpack your route. You can also gather information related to ideal weather windows on trail organization websites

and in online hiking forums specific to the trail you plan to hike. Keep in mind that these are just estimates. Seasonal variation, your skill and fitness level, and personal preference will determine what's appropriate for you.

Direction of Travel

The direction you decide to hike (northbound, southbound, eastbound, or westbound) also factors into your start date and affects the amount of solitude you'll experience on trail. Due to the climate and weather factors discussed, your chosen direction of travel will influence your choice of start date. Generally speaking, northbound hikers start in early spring once snow has melted at higher elevations in the south, and southbound hikers start a few months later once snow has melted in the north. On the Triple Crown trails (AT, PCT, and CDT), it's common for most people to hike northbound, so if you're seeking a highly social experience, plan to hike north during peak season. Southbound or shoulder-season travel will likely be a more solitary experience.

Permits

Permit availability also impacts your route choice, start date, and direction of travel. Some trails require a permit to hike legally and others don't. Check with trail organizations and state or federal land managers' websites for permit

BUDGETING

Lack of funds is one of the most common reasons that people either don't embark on their journey in the first place or leave the trail before finishing their hike. With a solid understanding of your finances, you can create a budget for your hike to determine how much you need to set aside for your desired adventure. If you need to save up, determine how long that will take you. You may hear estimates on how much to budget, such as $2 per mile or $1000 per month, but ultimately your expenses will depend on you.

Common expenses to factor into your budget include new gear, replacement gear, food for resupply, food and drink in town, lodging in town, and health insurance. Don't forget to include any expenses you'll still be paying at home, such as rent and cell phone bills. This list is not exhaustive and your budget will be unique to you.

I am able to complete long hikes for a fraction of what others spend by planning ahead, mailing resupply boxes, and rarely staying in towns. This is my preferred style. I invest my finances in the healthy foods that power me up the trail, and whenever I want a restaurant meal or hotel stay, it's in the budget. More often than not, though, I prefer to sleep in the woods and keep my town stays short. When creating your budget, know yourself and what best suits your preferences.

requirements and reservation methods for your chosen route. For many trails, permits are limited and assigned based on a lottery system, which may require you to apply more than six months in advance. Once you have your dates set for your hike, apply for permits and visas as soon as possible to lock in your spot. Have alternate dates in mind and be prepared to apply multiple times.

Who: Assembling Your Team

While it's certainly possible to plan and complete a long-distance hike by yourself, gathering a team can simplify logistics and improve the overall enjoyment of your hike. Your support team may be made up of those who hike along with you, your loved ones providing support from home, a point person to facilitate execution of your resupply strategy, and the broader hiking community.

Hiking Solo versus with Partners

Do you prefer to hike solo or with a partner or group? The majority of the long-distance hiking I have completed has been solo. I love the freedom, flexibility, and self-growth of backpacking

Heather Tip

If you're in a committed relationship or marriage and your partner will not be accompanying you on your hike, invest a lot of your planning and preparation time in preparing that relationship along with preparing for the hike itself. Each relationship is unique and there is no one way to navigate the problems that may arise from being apart and from reintegrating back into one another's lives afterward. Open communication is crucial—in the planning stage, on the trail, and after. You and your partner may even consider the benefit of working with a professional to facilitate the conversations throughout the entire process.

alone. I know many hikers, however, who prefer to hike with one or more partners for some or all of the trail; they like the camaraderie and support. There are pros and cons to each approach and it's important to know what works best for you.

A key component in deciding whether you will backpack solo or with a partner is understanding your individual risk tolerance. In terms of safety, solo backpacking is inherently less safe. If you do decide to travel alone, recognize the increased risks you'll be taking and plan for them. See chapter 3 for more about safety considerations. Despite the increased risk, solo backpacking is common, and it can be an incredibly rewarding experience that allows you to challenge yourself and develop greater self-reliance. When backpacking alone, you make all the decisions—and that is both a freedom and a responsibility.

Backpacking with a partner is not only the safer option but it can also be a great opportunity for bonding. It allows you to share gear, such as a tent or stove. It also requires more foresight, coordination, and patience. With every decision, each person's experience level, fitness, and preferences need to be taken into consideration.

On long trails with a strong social atmosphere, such as the AT and PCT, it's not uncommon for hikers to embark on their trip solo and meet hiking partners along the way. Some hikers stick

Hiking partners enjoy a sunset together at the end of a long day.

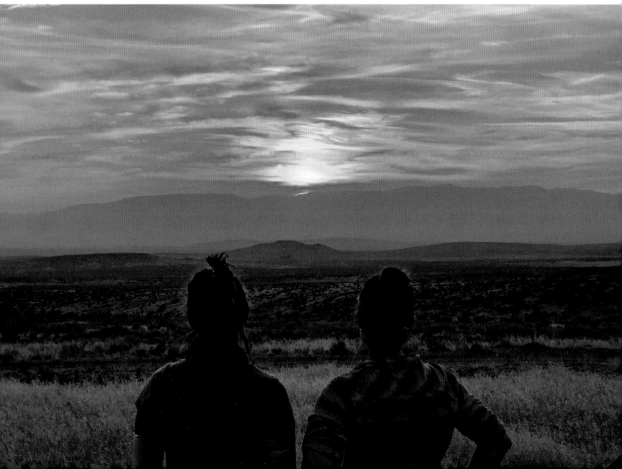

with their "trail family" for the entire hike. Others drift in and out of different groups. The latter was my approach on the AT and PCT. I appreciated the companionship of having a hiking partner for certain segments of the trail while maintaining the freedom to hike ahead or stay behind at my leisure.

Communicating Expectations with Your Hiking Partner

If you decide to hike with a partner, romantic or otherwise, it's important to discuss hiking styles and expectations in advance. Talk about your intentions for the trip, daily mileage goals, how you prefer to structure your day, how much time you like to spend in town, your budget, your risk tolerance, how much alone time you need, and how committed you are to sticking together for the entire trip.

Bypassing this step is a common mistake and can result in frustration, at best, and fractured relationships, at worst. I made this mistake on one of my early backpacking trips with a friend from high school. We had day-hiked but had never gone on a longer trip together. We were both too inexperienced to know that we should have discussed our expectations before setting foot on the trail. Because we failed to discuss our hiking styles and goals ahead of time, we both became frustrated and ended up parting ways during the multi-week hike. It was a difficult lesson to learn and it took many months to repair our friendship.

Hiking a long trail with another person has the potential to both bring you closer than ever and drive you completely apart. I've seen everything from trail marriages to breakups. Know that hiking a long trail brings out every aspect of you, and whoever you hike with will also experience your highest highs and lowest lows with you. There will be times when you're exhausted, hungry, walking through a rainstorm at dusk, with horrible blisters, and unable to find a suitable

Heather Tip

Not all families will be supportive, even if they're involved in the process. Many hikers, myself included, deal with a lot of negative familial pressure when preparing for their hikes. As with a romantic partner staying home, open communication is best. However, if the other parties cannot be open and continue to bully, make demands, or impose guilt, you may need to establish clear boundaries. Unfortunately, this can be a damaging process to the relationships, so take the time to be very honest with yourself about your needs and priorities and what you'll need to do to take care of yourself emotionally.

campsite. No matter how calm you are in your home environment, the trail will test you. Those are the times that it can be the hardest to show up as your "best self." Discuss with your hiking partner how you'll handle disagreements. Do your best to practice patience, compassion, and grace with each other.

Gathering Support at Home

As you formulate your trip plans, include the important people in your life in the process. When they understand exactly what you're doing and why, they can share in your excitement. Reassure them that you've thought through the details. You may wish to include them in the journey by requesting their support, either in the preparation phase or once you're on trail. Most likely, they'll feel excited to support you if they understand why your trip matters to you and they see that you're well prepared.

When I was planning my first long hike, I felt totally alone in the process, as if no one really understood what I was doing or why. Eventually, I realized I hadn't fully communicated my plans and excitement to my loved ones. Leaving them in the dark created concern on their part and a sense of feeling unsupported on my part. Once I shared how much the endeavor mattered to me

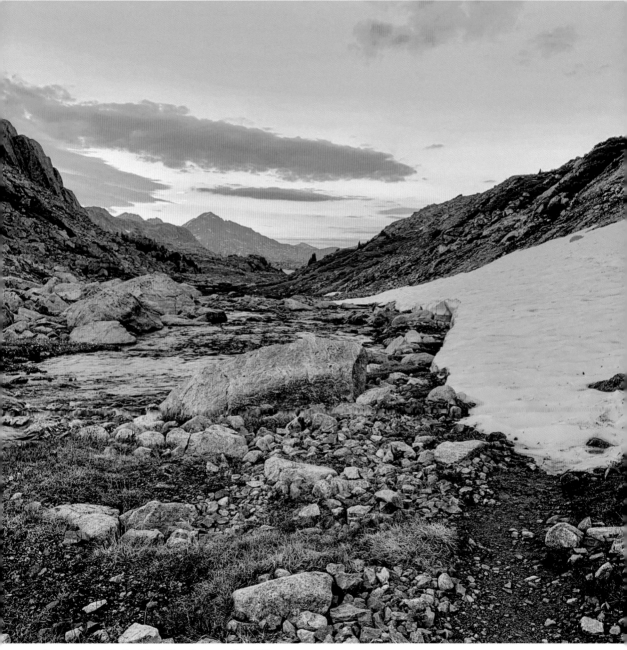

Dreamy sunset in the Wind River Range on the CDT

and that I was well prepared (or so I thought), their nerves were calmed and they became my biggest champions. I now have cherished memories of my parents helping me pack resupply boxes and of receiving letters and care packages from friends as I hiked up the trail, all as a result of inviting them into my planning process.

Choosing a Point Person

When hiking a long trail, you may wish to recruit a point person at home who is willing to support you while you're on trail. This person can be key to your success and can also serve as an emergency contact. Seek out someone reliable and organized, as you will likely depend on them heavily and you'll need to be in regular contact with the person, updating them on your progress and needs. Make your request for support months in advance of your hike, be explicit with what you're asking, and don't pressure them.

The primary duty of the point person is to mail your resupply boxes and extra gear to you on trail. Make their job easier and your trip more enjoyable by leaving clear instructions and having resupply boxes and extra gear organized, packed, and labeled before you go so that your point person only needs to close the boxes and drop them at the post office. Along with your itinerary, include instructions for whom to contact in case of an emergency and provide key phone numbers (vet, landlord, family) and passwords. Leave spare keys and cash (or blank checks) for unexpected expenses. You may even wish to give someone at home power of attorney to make legal decisions for you while you're on trail. Consider what could possibly go wrong and plan ahead.

While you don't absolutely need a point person, having one takes a lot of stress off of you during your hike. The longer the hike, the more helpful this can be. At minimum, and even on shorter hikes, leave your itinerary with someone at home and provide clear instructions on what to do if you don't check in when you're expected. And remember that your point person is your MVP, so treat them as such: shower them with love and praise often.

Connecting with the Hiking Community

Connecting with the hiking community online and in person before your hike is an excellent way to get excited and help you prepare. Relating to others who have achieved the goal you're going after reminds you that you're not alone in your aspirations and that you're capable. Experienced backpackers can offer a wealth of information and answer questions ranging from gear selection to how to properly poop in the woods.

If you're new to backpacking and don't personally know any experienced backpackers, search platforms such as Meetup.com for local groups, take outdoor skill courses, and attend events like the annual spring Rucks (workshops designed to prepare backpackers for the trail) hosted by the American Long-Distance Hiking Association-West (see Additional Resources). There are also myriad outdoors groups on platforms such as Facebook and Reddit. Reading hiking-related memoirs and listening to hiking podcasts can also help you feel connected to the community and bring the dream alive before you even set foot on trail.

RESEARCHING LIKELY CONDITIONS

Once you've finalized when, where, and with whom you're going, familiarize yourself with your chosen route and assess the conditions you're likely to encounter. This sets the stage to create an itinerary, plan your gear, assemble a resupply plan, and evaluate and mitigate risk. It also provides you with a better understanding of how to prepare physically and mentally.

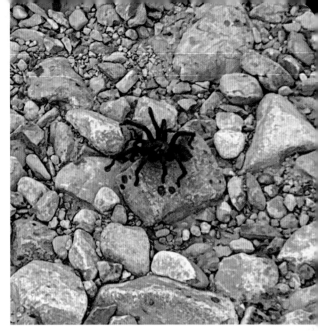

A tarantula in an arroyo near the Mexican border on the CDT

In this stage of planning, you'll want to reevaluate the weather and climate for your destination as well as the topography and trail type. In addition, research route conditions, such as the necessary navigational tools, where the water sources will be, possible wildlife encounters, how remote the route is, and whether any restrictions or closures may be in effect during your trip.

What follows are questions, or prompts, to help guide your research into each set of conditions. Some of these trip conditions may not exist on every route and there may be others you wish to include that aren't on this list. Consult chapters 3 and 4, on backcountry safety and navigation, to learn more about each of these risk factors and how to create a personalized preparation plan for your chosen route.

Seasons, Climate, and Weather

What season(s) will you be hiking in? How much daylight will there be? Based on your earlier research, what is the expected climate and weather? What are the averages for precipitation and temperature? What are the record highs and lows? As you get closer to your trip dates, remember to check the weather forecast.

Terrain

Terrain refers to the physical features of the land, such as mountains, forests, or floodplains. What types of terrain will you encounter? How much of your route is above tree line? How much of your route is forested? What is the degree of sun exposure, or the extent of elevation gain and loss?

Trail Type

Consider the type of trail on which you'll be hiking. Will it be a well-marked and maintained trail or will you be hiking off trail? Will you be traveling across scree or boulder fields? Is there vegetation? If so, what type, and do you need special gear/clothing to avoid spiny or poisonous plants? Does your route require scrambling or climbing? Will you encounter year-round or glaciated snow, and if so, how much?

Navigation

What navigational tools do you need? Do you have an understanding of the broader area beyond just the trail you're hiking? Are you familiar with alternate routes and potentially confusing junctions? If you were to go off route, where are the closest roads? What prominent landmarks, such as mountains or rivers, can you look for?

Water Sources and Obstacles

Where are the water sources along your route, and are they likely to be flowing at your chosen time of year? What is the source (spring, stream, river, lake, etc.)? Is the source directly on your route or will you need to hike off trail to find it? Are there river crossings? How wide and deep do you expect them to be?

Wildlife Interactions

What animals are you likely to encounter on this route? What are the risks? How will you deal with the situation if you encounter any of these animals?

Human Interactions and Remoteness

Are you likely to encounter other humans on this route? How remote is the route? How likely will it be for someone to find you if you're injured? Where are the nearest roads? How will you be evacuated in case of an emergency?

Restrictions and Closures

Are there any fire restrictions? Will you encounter any sections of trail that may be closed due to events like a downed bridge, wildfire or natural disaster, or for species restoration?

As you evaluate each of these factors and plan your trip, order and print any maps, data books, and guidebooks you will need for your hike in both digital and paper formats. Other resources that can assist you in finding the most up-to-date conditions include trip reports, online forums, land managers, trail association websites, historical weather data, backcountry

rangers, and experienced backcountry users. These are all excellent sources to draw upon in the creation of your beta packet (see chapter 4).

CREATING YOUR ITINERARY

When I "planned" that first AT hike, I didn't create an itinerary at all. It didn't even occur to me to do so, and if it had, I wouldn't have known where to start. This failure resulted in frustration for my point person, wasted money on hotel rooms (while waiting for resupply boxes), miscalculated food needs, and just more stress than was necessary.

Creating an itinerary for your trip allows you to plan campsites, secure permits, determine how much food to pack, and to communicate your plans with hiking partners and your emergency contact person. Key variables to consider are your route length, expected daily mileage, and start and end dates. For a shorter trip, create a day-to-day itinerary in terms of mileage goals and campsites. For a longer trip, there's no need to plan your itinerary down to the day as it's highly unusual for long-distance hikers to adhere to a preplanned itinerary on a multi-week or multi-month trip. However, creating a broad

SAMPLE ITINERARY				
DATE	LOCATION	CUMULATIVE SOUTHBOUND MILES	MILES OFF TRAIL (ONE-WAY)	MILES TO NEXT RESUPPLY
JUNE	MONTANA			
17	Chief Mountain	0	on trail	91.2
20	East Glacier	91.2	on trail	177
27	Lincoln	268.2	20 miles W	68.6
30	Helena	336.8	15 miles E	74.4
JULY				
3	Anaconda	411.2	on trail	91.2

itinerary for a long hike is helpful so you can plan your resupply and know your daily mileage targets to ensure you finish by your projected end date.

It may seem tedious (or exciting, depending on your love of spreadsheets), but the process outlined here provides an estimate of how long it will take you to finish the trail and gives you a clear idea of how much time you can spend in towns along the way and still finish before your projected end date. You may find that you need to set your daily mileage goals higher so that you finish in time. Or you may decide that based on your current mileage abilities and the length of your chosen route that you want to break your trip into sections to be completed over multiple hiking seasons.

A spreadsheet is also ideal for itinerary creation so that you can keep data organized and make adjustments easily. There are online planners, such as Craig's PCT Planner (see Additional Resources), that can help you understand how variables such as terrain affect your daily mileage. It can be a useful exercise to play with one of these calculators to wrap your mind around planning a hiking schedule.

Determining Daily Mileage

When estimating your daily mileage, ask yourself: What distance am I *certain* I can comfortably hike in a day? Take into consideration your current fitness level and past experiences and the elevation gain and terrain type for your route. When traveling with a group, determine daily mileage estimates based on the slowest member of the group. Be conservative in your estimates.

Especially on shorter routes, consider available daylight and whether you'll want to hike in the dark. Waking up with the sun at five to hike on a warm July morning is a much different experience than crawling out of your sleeping bag at the same time on a chilly October morning to hike in the dark for a few hours.

On a longer trip, break your itinerary into shorter segments based on resupply points to make it easier to make projections. To determine how many days it will take you to get from one resupply point to the next, calculate the distance (in miles) between point A and point B. Divide that distance by your expected daily mileage for that leg of the trip. The result is the number of days you should plan to complete that section

BUY IN TOWN OR MAIL	NUMBER OF DAYS OF FOOD AT 25 MILES PER DAY	PO BOX AND MAIL-DROP INFO AND ADDRESS
grocery	3.6	
USPS	7.1	Hiker c/o Brownies Hostel, 1020 Montana Hwy 49, East Glacier Park, MT 59434
USPS	2.7	Hiker c/o Three Bears Motel, PO Box 995, Lincoln, MT 59639
USPS	3	Hiker c/o Budget Inn Express, 524 N Last Chance Gulch, Helena, MT 59601
grocery	3.4	

of trail. You can also use that number to plan the amount of food to purchase for that section or to include in your resupply box if you're sending one. Move on to the next segment and repeat the calculation until you have an estimated number of days for your entire trip.

It's also recommended that you plan "zero days" (days where you do not hike while staying in town or at a beautiful spot on trail) and add buffer days into your itinerary in case you move slower or faster than expected, which is quite likely: your daily mileage is bound to increase over the course of a long trip as you get your "trail legs." Update your itinerary as you go and keep your point person informed.

There are a number of factors, such as terrain, trail type, weather, altitudes, backpack weight, and elevation gain that affect daily mileage. It's highly dependent on the route and the hiker, but I generally estimate a 50 percent increase in mileage (e.g. from 20 miles per day to 30 miles per day) after about 300 miles of a trip, while remembering to factor in buffer days for difficult terrain, off-trail travel, and town stops. Your estimates may look very different from mine; use your past experiences to find what works for you. For more detailed strategies to help you plan daily mileage for your trip, turn to chapter 7.

Considering Trip Preferences

Another component of planning your daily mileage is to decide how many hours you want to hike each day. What ratio of hiking to camping do you prefer? Do you want to hike all day, get to camp at dusk, eat, sleep, and be out of camp at sunrise? Or do you prefer to hike a few hours of the day and spend more time relaxing in camp? Decide where you fall along that spectrum. On a longer trip, you will most likely need to be hiking for a greater portion of the day in order to finish the trail. On shorter trips, you have more leeway.

Campsite Selection

Planning specific campsites for a long trail is not recommended since dates invariably shift on long-distance hikes. Rather, it's helpful to know *how* to select a campsite so that each evening in your tent, you can review your route for the next day, evaluate the topography, take into account your daily mileage goals, and get a general sense for where you'll camp the following day. You may not always get there, but having a daily goal can help you stick to your broad itinerary.

Note that there may be certain segments of your trip, such as when traveling through national parks, where you will need to apply for permits and stay in preselected campsites. Otherwise, you can use the following guidelines for campsite selection.

In general, choose sites that are not at the lowest or highest point in an area. This helps you avoid cold valleys and windy ridges. Steer clear of low-lying water, which attracts bugs and cold-settling air. Avoid areas prone to flash floods, such as drainages, and do not set up under dead trees (a.k.a. widow-makers) that could fall in the night. Finding a spot that is secluded, protected by sturdy trees, and with soft, durable ground cover, such as pine duff, is ideal. Selecting campsites within a relatively short distance of a water source is convenient for cooking and rehydrating at the end/beginning of the day.

Camping Responsibly

To reduce your impact in the backcountry, camp on durable surfaces that will withstand wear, such as rock, sand, or gravel. This is Leave No Trace principle no. 2 (see "The Seven Principles of Leave No Trace" sidebar in chapter 2). When selecting a campsite, consider the frequency of use in the area, the fragility of the vegetation and soil, the likelihood of wildlife disturbance, and your group's potential to cause impact. Avoid camping close to trails and within 200 feet of water to allow access routes

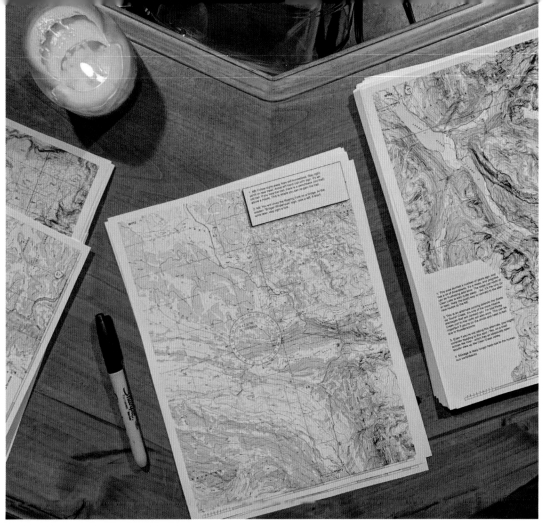

Studying maps in preparation for a thru-hike

for wildlife. Obey any local regulations related to campsite selection. In high-use areas, choose campsites that are so highly impacted that careful use will cause no further noticeable impact, such as a site that has already lost its vegetation. Similarly, traffic routes and kitchens should be located in already highly impacted areas.

When camping in undisturbed remote areas, the approach is different: Spread out campsites and avoid using the same routes to water, the cooking area, and any other common areas. Watch where you walk to avoid crushing vegetation and walking on sensitive surfaces, such as living soil or lichen. When leaving a remote campsite, take time to naturalize the site. Cover areas with native materials, rake matted grass with a stick, and brush out footprints. Make it less likely for other backcountry travelers to camp in the same spot so that the site remains in good condition.

Distributing Your Itinerary

Create a copy of your itinerary to take with you. Leave copies with friends and family, including your point person, so that they know when and where to send resupply boxes, letters, or care packages. I keep a digital version on my phone as well. In addition to dates, resupply points, addresses, phone numbers, and important notes, include contact information for local emergency personnel and leave instructions such as "If I'm not back by this date, this is who you need to contact." On shorter hikes, include intended campsites. You may also want to include descriptions and photos of your gear (see Itinerary & Emergency Contact Worksheet in Worksheets & Checklists at the back of the book).

Booking Your Transportation and Lodging

As soon as you set your start date, determine exactly how you will get to the trailhead so that you can arrange transportation and pre-trip lodging if needed. Keep in mind that you may need to arrange multiple legs of the journey. For instance, if you are flying, arrange for ground transportation from the airport to the trailhead. If you are taking a bus, shuttle, or train, be sure you know the schedule, fares, and drop-off location as well as how you will get to the trailhead from that point.

Be sure to take potential delays into account, especially if the journey involves multiple legs, and even more so if your chosen form of transport is not 100 percent reliable (e.g., hitchhiking). When I hiked the CDT southbound, my journey just to reach the northern terminus at the Canadian border in Glacier National Park required multiple pieces: First, I flew into Kalispell, Montana. A friend then picked me up and drove me to Glacier National Park so that I could get my permit. From there, I hitchhiked up to my starting point.

You likely won't have to start from scratch with your research. If you plan to hike a popular trail, search trail organization websites, trip reports, and hiker forums online to find your options for getting to the trailhead. In some areas, hiker shuttles offer transportation to and from trailheads, as do "trail angels"—people who help hikers by offering food, lodging, transportation, and other acts of kindness and generosity. Book early as shuttles often fill up quickly, especially during peak hiker season.

For shorter trips, if you drive to the trailhead, plan accordingly: Look up the directions in advance, and print or save them to a note on your phone in case you lose service on the way. If you're going with a group, decide who will be driving. Research expected road conditions and trailhead parking. Determine if you need a four-wheel drive vehicle. Seek out the most up-to-date information from trip reports, online maps, and by contacting regional Forest Service offices.

SELECTING YOUR GEAR

Once you've defined the parameters of your trip and created an itinerary, it's time to select and gather your gear! Acquiring the appropriate gear for your route is an essential element of safe and enjoyable backcountry travel. A well-organized gear list allows you to calculate pack weight and track costs and can also be used as a pre-departure checklist and a packing template for future trips.

While proper gear can make or break your trip, many hikers get unnecessarily tripped up on this step, spending excess time, money, and stress creating the "perfect" gear list. A brief internet search reveals no shortage of options and opinions, making it easy to fall down a rabbit hole during this part of the trip-planning process. This can lead to stress and feeling overwhelmed. But it doesn't need to be this way. Approach this part of the planning process with greater ease by using your expected route conditions to inform your choices and remembering that you can swap out items along the way. For an in-depth exploration of gear selection and sample gear lists, refer to chapter 2; this section briefly discusses the factors that influence gear selection as they relate to trip planning.

Factors That Influence Gear Selection

Your gear choices will be shaped by the trip conditions you outlined earlier as well as by your experience level and personal preferences. Carrying the appropriate gear for your trip allows you to travel comfortably and safely and helps you avoid carrying "just in case" items, because you know what the likely conditions will be. Review the expected conditions for your route to evaluate how each impacts your gear choices.

The data you gather regarding season, climate, and weather will obviously affect many of your gear choices. For example, expected temperatures influence sleeping bag and clothing choices; expected precipitation affects your choice of raingear and gear protection; and expected snow travel will determine whether you carry microspikes.

Another element to consider is the likelihood of potential animal encounters. Choices you make here could include: carrying an odor-proof sack to protect your food from mice, chipmunks, and other rodents; carrying insect repellent and bug netting if you're expecting heavy bug pressure; or carrying an Ursack or bear canister for storing your food if you'll be in bear country or in an area where backpackers are required to carry a bear canister.

Again, gear selection should be specific to the route conditions you expect to encounter. Creating a template and referencing other gear lists—especially for trips in similar locations—can be helpful, but avoid blindly copying someone else's gear list without personalizing it for your chosen route and preferences.

If you want additional feedback on your gear list, ask an experienced backpacker to evaluate your list or post it to a backpacking forum, such as Ultralight Reddit or a Facebook backpacking group. There will be no shortage of opinions. Consider the background and experience level of anyone giving you advice and trust your own experience above all else. Make conservative

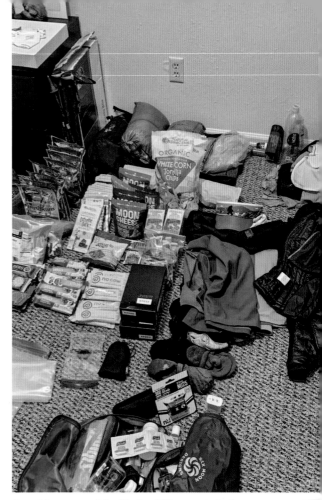

Organizing gear and food before hiking a route in the Great Basin

choices and do what's most appropriate for the conditions of your chosen route.

Once you know what gear you will need for your trip, take inventory of what you and any hiking partners already have and what you will need to acquire. Decide what you will buy or borrow, if anything. For the items you already own, inspect their condition. If an item is damaged, such as a broken tent pole or ripped tarp, replace it or repair it. Newly acquired and borrowed items should be tested before your trip commences if possible. See chapter 2 for more information on acquiring borrowed or used gear and on testing your gear.

If you plan to hike with a hiking partner, sharing gear allows you to distribute the weight of certain items so that each person can reduce their pack weight. Shared items might include a tent, a stove, or a cooking pot. If you decide to share gear with a hiking partner, be sure each member of the group is committed to staying together for the duration of the trip.

PLANNING YOUR FOOD RESUPPLY STRATEGY

"What am I going to eat?!"

This is a big concern for hikers heading out on a long backpacking trip. If you're hiking a long trail that requires you to resupply along the way, planning a resupply strategy before you go allows you to know when and where you will pick up your next food drop. The complexity of your resupply strategy will be related to the complexity of your chosen route and your personal preferences. If you're hiking a well-traveled, easily accessible route such as the AT, you may not need much of a resupply strategy. If, on the other hand, you're traveling a route through a remote region where resupply options are slim, your strategy will be more robust. To resupply food and fuel needs on trail, there are a few options:

1. Prepare boxes in advance and ask a point person to mail them to you on trail.
2. Buy food as you go and mail boxes ahead to yourself as needed.
3. Employ a mix of strategies 1 and 2.

Each of these strategies begins with identifying potential resupply locations along your route. You can find this information by looking at your maps, consulting trail organization websites, and reviewing other hikers' blogs. Once you identify potential resupply locations, evaluate the available grocery options and determine if the selection meets your needs. If not, plan to send a box to that location, either by having your point person send it or by mailing it yourself from a town with more grocery options earlier on your route. For example, I hike best when I eat healthy food, so if I identify a resupply location where the only grocery option is a gas station, I'll send myself a box to that town.

Strategy 1: Prepare Resupply Boxes in Advance

This strategy requires that you purchase all of your food in advance, repackage it, box it up before you hit the trail, and recruit a responsible point person to send your boxes out in a timely fashion to the towns en route where you determine you need or want a box.

The best approach is to pack and address your boxes ahead of time but do not tape them shut; your point person may need to add or subtract items before mailing. You might also consider numbering your boxes so that you can instruct your point person to "please send box #3 out by X date." That way, your point person doesn't have to do any guesswork. Make it easy for them!

Pros

- Guarantee your nutritional needs, wants, and desires are met. Great for those who prefer organic, have dietary restrictions, or need prescription medications.
- You can budget your food.
- Avoid spending time in town purchasing food for the next stretch. This frees up time to relax, or you may opt to pick up your box and pass through without needing to pay for lodging. This option is good if you're in a hurry.
- You can send hard-to-find items, such as gas for your stove (via ground shipping only).
- If there's an item you discover you need while on trail, you can ask your point person to send it.

- You can add your maps to your food box to avoid mailing them separately or having to carry all of them.

Cons

- You're stuck eating what's in your box unless you give it away and purchase food in town, which is not recommended if you're on a budget.
- Requires more planning time before you hit the trail.
- Post office hours vary and sometimes you may get into town after the post office is closed or on a Sunday, requiring that you wait until the following morning to get your food.
- The box may get sent back if it isn't picked up in time.
- The delivery timing could get mixed up by your point person or just fail to reach your pickup location.

Strategy 2: Buy As You Go

If you don't have dietary restrictions or preferences and you want to ease the prep time before you embark on your adventure, you may opt to buy as you go. Although most towns have grocery stores where you can purchase food, some may have only a gas station/convenience store, which is less than ideal when it comes to nutrition. For locations with limited options, identify a town with good resupply options that you'll be passing through at least ten days before you plan to be at the location with limited options. Plan to buy extra food in the well-stocked town and mail it ahead to the location with limited options. Mailing your box at least ten days in advance ensures enough time for your box to reach the next location before you do. This strategy requires that you have an estimate of your daily mileage.

Pros

- You can purchase food you are craving and change up your menu as you hike.
- If you have food left over when getting into town, you save money by not buying those items.
- You're not tethered to the business hours of the post office.
- You get to support local businesses.
- If you have to leave the trail for any reason, you don't have leftover trail food boxed up at home.

Cons

- Prices can be higher than average in remote stores.
- Organic, vegetarian, vegan, gluten-free, and other specialty items are not as widely available in small towns.
- On popular trails, hikers ahead of you may wipe out staple items before you arrive.

Strategy 3: The Combined Approach

Many hikers use a combination of both strategies. This entails sending resupply boxes from home or ahead to oneself on trail as well as purchasing from grocery stores in well-stocked towns. This strategy works well because it offers the best of the first two strategies. It ensures that any hard-to-find items are provided while also offering variety and spontaneity. Shipping prepurchased items to places where resupply options are more expensive and purchasing in towns where prices are more moderate saves money overall.

How to Send a Box When One Is Needed

Plan for mail to take at least five to seven days. If you're mailing from the trail, use your daily mileage to calculate how many miles you'll cover

From: (return address)

> Jane Hiker
> General Delivery
> Town, State Zip

Please Hold for Jane Hiker, **ETA:** Date

Write "PLEASE HOLD FOR (hiker name), ETA: (date)" somewhere on the outside of the box and always include a return address.

during that time, and plan accordingly so your box reaches your destination before you do. If a point person is mailing your box, instruct them to send it at least ten days before you want to receive it. A popular option for mailing food drops is to use flat rate boxes sent via General Delivery to United States Post Service offices. Most post offices will hold General Delivery boxes for two weeks. Alternatively, outfitters, hostels, and motels in trail towns often accept hiker boxes as well. With either option, call ahead to confirm the address and hours. If it's not a post office, ask whether they'll hold your box and if there's a fee.

How to Pack and Protect Your Food On Trail

When packing your food, remove as much packaging as possible. This reduces bulk in your pack as well as the amount of waste that you need to pack out. Protect food by carrying an odor-proof sack to prevent mice and other rodents from eating your food in the nighttime. Carry a bear canister or Ursack in bear country. For detailed information on calculating food needs, maximizing backcountry nutrition for optimal performance, and creating an ultralight, healthy backcountry meal plan, see chapter 6.

SAFETY IN THE BACKCOUNTRY

Learning how to assess and prepare for potential risk factors in the backcountry is an essential component of planning a successful backpacking trip. This section is intended as an introduction to the topic of backcountry safety for the purposes of initial planning. For a thorough review of potential factors that may impact your safety in the backcountry, ways to mitigate those risks, and a framework for creating your own personalized backcountry preparation plan, see chapter 3.

Simply put, creating a backcountry preparation plan specific to your trip can save your life. When you are in an unfamiliar or stressful situation in the backcountry, your brain isn't thinking clearly and your decision-making ability is muddled. Waiting to think through a scenario until you're in a dangerous situation is too late. As they say: hope for the best and plan for the worst.

Heather Tip

Through trial and error, a combined approach has become my go-to. As someone with a dietary restriction, I know what I generally struggle to find on trail and what I don't, so I send either partial or full resupplies to locations where I know my choices will be limited. I do not have a point person at home, though, so I package and mail my boxes myself before I go out. This is an extra level of preparation because I have to ensure I don't forget things, but it also works well for me. I always double-check with any business I send a box to that they accept them and that they will hold it until I arrive. I also use a mailing service that provides tracking and keeps tabs on my packages so there aren't surprises.

● My system follows the 500-mile interval: Since I replace my shoes every 500 miles, I know I will send a box to locations at that interval with shoes in it. I often send extra items in that box that I can use to replace/replenish what I've been carrying or forward ahead if I don't need them yet (socks, first-aid supplies, etc.).

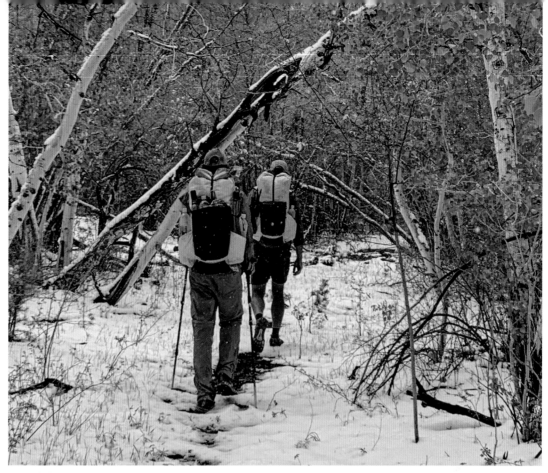

Hiking in inclement weather, such as this late spring storm in Nevada, is safer when you've planned for it and are prepared with proper gear and skills.

To evaluate possible risks specific to your trip, review conditions for your chosen route and consider how each could affect your safety. Contemplate every detail relevant to where you'll be hiking, and for each scenario, know how you would respond. For example, with weather conditions, what will happen if it's colder, hotter, or wetter than you expect? Are you prepared? What if you go off route, become injured, or have an adverse animal or human encounter? If you plan to hike in an area inhabited by grizzlies, such as Glacier National Park, do you know typical grizzly bear behavior and techniques to avoid encounters, especially if you're solo? Do you intend to carry bear spray, and is it attached to an easy-to-access area? Have you practiced unholstering the bear spray, unclipping it, and aiming?

Consider each risk factor and determine how you can prepare for that situation or avoid getting into that situation in the first place. Mitigation tactics may include carrying special gear relevant to the expected conditions, such as bear spray, microspikes, or additional warm layers. You also may need to expand your knowledge base and skill set. Proper preparation includes thinking ahead, planning, and acquiring the necessary knowledge, gear, and skills pertinent to your route.

TRIP-PLANNING CHECKLIST

- [ ] Finalize location: start and finish trailheads
- [ ] Finalize trip dates
- [ ] Acquire necessary permits and park passes
- [ ] Book transportation (airfare, ground transportation)
- [ ] Book pre- and post-trip lodging
- [ ] Coordinate with hiking partners
- [ ] Research likely route conditions
- [ ] Create itinerary
- [ ] Acquire navigational tools (maps, GPS tracks, data books, etc.)
- [ ] Develop and follow a physical training plan
- [ ] Make a gear list
- [ ] Inventory current gear, make repairs if necessary
- [ ] Acquire any gear items still needed
- [ ] Assemble first-aid kit
- [ ] Create a resupply plan
- [ ] Calculate food needs
- [ ] Purchase and package shelf-stable food
- [ ] Buy perishable food (a day before leaving)
- [ ] Leave a copy of itinerary and resupply information with emergency contact/point person
- [ ] Load map files to GPS unit or smartphone for offline use
- [ ] Set compass declination for the area where you're traveling
- [ ] Top off charge for all electronics, including battery backups
- [ ] Print permits
- [ ] Set up things on the homefront: arrange for house/pet/plant sitter, set bills to auto-pay, set email autoresponder, put mail on hold

PREPARING YOURSELF PHYSICALLY AND MENTALLY

Many hikers spend a disproportionate amount of time researching gear, planning their resupply, and reading trip reports—and while these components are critical to success, it's equally important to focus on the physical and mental preparation that can make or break an adventure.

Physical preparation involves fully preparing your body for the rigors of hiking through physical training and creating health resilience, thus reducing your chance of injury and illness and increasing the likelihood that your body can withstand months of walking ten or more hours per day. These topics are explored in greater detail in subsequent chapters: In chapter 5, learn strategies for gut health, sleep, and stress mitigation that will help you optimize your energy and endurance on trail. Chapter 7 guides you through creating a focused training plan prior to departure that will enable you to build strength and endurance, reducing the potential of developing overuse injuries on trail.

In addition to physical preparation, proper mental and emotional preparation is essential to the success of your journey. It's often said that "thru-hiking success is 90 percent mental." Chapter 8 discusses tools and techniques to help you prepare for the mental challenges of spending weeks or months traveling through the wilderness. Tasks covered earlier in this chapter—such as familiarizing yourself with your gear, creating your backcountry preparation plan, and researching your trip conditions—will also help you mentally prepare for a successful journey. Knowledge and preparation weigh nothing and could save your life.

THE FINAL CHECK

Before you embark on your big adventure, do a final check to be sure you have everything in order! Checklists are great for this. Give yourself plenty of time and don't wait until the night before you leave to be sure you're ready to go. Coordinate with your hiking partners ahead of time and more than once to be sure you're on the same page in terms of dates, transportation, and other key details.

At least a week or more before your departure, depending on the complexity of your trip, finalize your transportation and print your permits. Be sure you have your rides lined up for each leg of the journey. Check that you have directions saved to your phone. Double-check flight times and bus or shuttle schedules. Purchase, package, and prepare your food. If you're flying, you may want to wait until you arrive to purchase certain items like food, fuel, or bear spray that may be prohibited in carry-on or checked luggage. If you'll be gone for an extended period of time, be sure you've handled everything at home such as pet sitters, mail holding or forwarding, bill auto-pay, and so forth.

At least three to four days before departure, review your gear list and pack your pack. Check in with your trip partners (again!) to be sure everything is on schedule. Proofread your itinerary and share it with your point person/emergency contact if you haven't already done so. Double-check your navigation tools. Do you have a way to protect paper maps in the field? Have you set your compass declination for the area where you're traveling? Do you have the correct maps and overlays downloaded to your device for offline use? Have you downloaded a wider corridor, beyond your trail, so that you can find your way out in an emergency situation?

A day or two before you leave, be sure all your electronics are charged up, including your phone, external batteries, USB headlamps, GPS watch, and emergency satellite devices. Have your gear, clothes, permits, park pass, and food ready to go. Pack extra snacks, water, and comfy clothes and shoes for pre-trip travel, if needed. Go back over everything one last time and get a good night's rest before your big adventure!

2

GEAR SELECTION

BY *Katie & Heather*

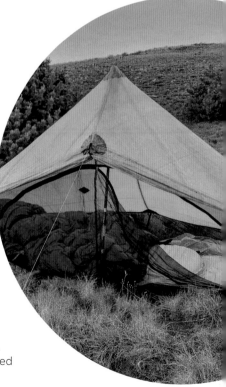

The most important thing to remember when choosing gear is that there is no one-size-fits-all gear list for every person in all conditions on all trails. Even as experienced backpackers, we still experiment with new items and mix and match from different gear lists on our trips! Neither of us is particularly "into" gear. We're not necessarily concerned with having the newest, lightest, or most popular piece of gear on the market. Neither of us follow gear trends at all. Yet between us, we've walked the equivalent of three laps around the equator successfully. Bear this in mind the next time you begin to feel like gear selection is the make-or-break issue when preparing for a long-distance journey!

In this chapter we cover the factors that influence gear selection for various types of trails and conditions as well as gear-specific issues of weight, durability, cost, etc. We also discuss what gear we personally use and why in order to give you a broader understanding of our personal selection process. With these tools, you'll be able to decide what you want and need from your gear and can begin to build your kit.

A word on choosing gear based on recommendations from online forums: know your source. First, consider the hiking experience and testing conditions the person used the gear in. Gear that they loved on the PCT might not work well on the AT, for example. Second, this is the only time it's recommended to compare yourself directly with someone else! In all seriousness, the gear items that work for me (Heather)—a 5-foot-7, middle-aged woman—are probably not going to be the best options for a twenty-two-year-old 6-foot-4, man. Look for people who are physically similar to you, who hike similarly to you (how much time do they walk each day compared to tent time?), and on similar terrain. The closer the comparison, the more likely a recommendation is going to work for you.

ROUTE CONDITIONS

While many of our base pieces remain the same across conditions, we swap many supporting parts out depending on the anticipated route conditions. Where you are hiking and on what type of surface dramatically impacts the gear you choose to take with you on a given trip. When you base your gear selection on expected route conditions, you reduce the likelihood that you will pack items "just in case," such as an extra shirt or down pants because you don't know what temperature range to expect. As mentioned, the gear you use on the PCT may vary wildly from that which you'd use on the AT. Even over the course of the PCT, you may find that you need different items as you progress from arid California to drizzly Washington. Similarly, the footwear appropriate for a long trip through the Rockies may not be as ideal for a journey through the Ouachitas.

As discussed in chapter 1, it's important to research your trail prior to setting out. Not only can it increase your safety but it will help you make informed choices about gear options. Your gear choices will be influenced by the type of trail tread likely to be encountered, altitude of the route and extent of tree cover, remoteness, possible animal encounters, local food-storage regulations, as well as the climate and weather.

Rocky trails and off-trail travel may require more durable footwear and trekking poles. High routes with considerable scrambling may require stiffer, more fitted footwear. High-altitude hiking may require more fuel (and food!). Wide-open hiking, such as in the desert, may require the use of a sun umbrella or higher-coverage hat and clothes. If bears inhabit portions of your route, you may wish to carry bear spray, and local regulations may require that you store food in a bear canister. When hiking in peak mosquito season, you may wish to carry a head net and bug netting for your shelter if it is not included already.

WEATHER

Weather makes a huge difference on the trail because, unlike at home, you can't escape it aside from getting into your shelter—which you've hopefully selected based on the climate of your route!

When evaluating how weather will influence your gear selection, refer to the trip-planning research you did (see chapter 1). Look at seasonal averages for temperature and precipitation to inform your choices. Adjust for elevation by assuming a 3- to 5-degree drop in temperature for every 1000 feet of elevation gain. Use this data to make decisions about sleeping bag

> **Heather Tip**
>
> *My thru-hikes of the Oregon Desert Trail and CDT in 2017 had resupply points spaced as much as eight days (240 miles) apart! I used a backpack that was an additional 25 liters in capacity over what I used on the AT fastest known time (FKT) in 2015, where my average resupply was every two and a half days (100 miles).*

ratings, clothing and layering options, raingear, and items like microspikes and sun umbrellas.

Weather isn't just about the number of rainy days or average temperatures. Things like humidity and wind can also influence your choices. Seasonality also plays a role. For example, when I (Heather) hiked the Calendar-Year Triple Crown in 2018, I traversed the Appalachian Mountains in very early spring. Rather than hot, humid, soggy conditions, which are the standard in the summer, I hiked through snow day after day in temperatures hovering around freezing. My clothing and gear choices looked more like

they do for winter mountaineering in the Pacific Northwest. I wore many layers, carried a larger backpack, thicker sleeping pad, down booties, and waterproof socks.

From there I went over to the New Mexico portion of the CDT and then on to the PCT. I completely overhauled my gear before I hopped on the plane from New Hampshire to Albuquerque. Instead of cold and snow, I transitioned into hot, exposed, and dry conditions. My water-storage capacity quadrupled, sleeping bag went from a rating of 0 degrees to 45, and my insulated skirt, tights, mid-top shoes, and

Oregon Desert Trail vista (Photo by Whitney LaRuffa)

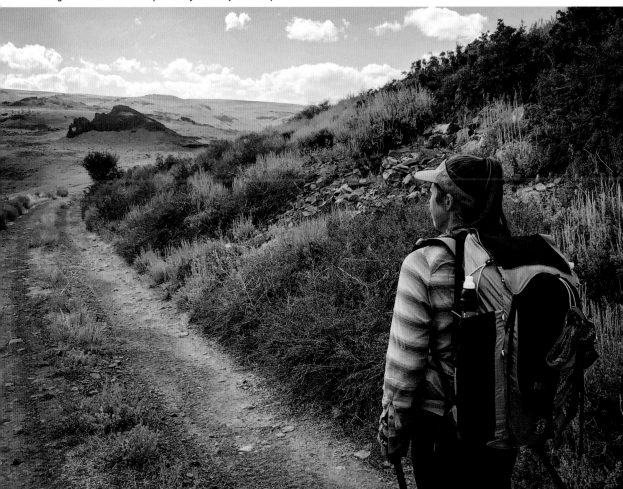

knee-high gaiters were swapped out for low-cut trail runners, shorts, and a sun umbrella!

RESUPPLY AND WATER ACCESS FREQUENCY

Resupply frequency (and type of resupply available) will primarily influence your pack type and size, as well as your choice of food preparation. As you develop your strategy for resupplying, you will get a stronger sense of the capacity requirements of your backpack. A good rule of thumb is to choose the pack that will work for 95 percent of the projected resupplies. It's usually not worth it to carry a lot of empty backpack most of the time when you can just strap bags of chips or a bear canister onto the outside of a smaller pack for the few days that space is a concern.

Your access to water is also a determining factor for pack capacity. On very dry trails such as the Arizona Trail, you may need to carry the same capacity backpack you use for longer food-carry hikes, even if you have shorter resupply intervals. Water takes up a lot of space inside your backpack, in addition to being heavy. In the gear-list portion of this chapter, we share our specific gear choices and notes on why we chose some of them.

EVALUATING, CHOOSING, AND TESTING GEAR

The best method for evaluating whether a particular piece of gear works for you is to use it in the field. Nothing is more telling than a few days

> **Heather Tip**
> While I am just on the fringe of ultralight (my base weight is 9 to 12 pounds), the concept of choosing the lightest piece that will function for me is prevalent in my decision-making. This helps ensure that my pack weight doesn't swell out of control (except with food!).

> **Katie Tip**
> I began my first long-distance hike with a thrifted external-frame backpack, a 4-pound sleeping bag, and several pieces of borrowed gear. My pack weighed 55 pounds! Slogging up and down those mountains in the first 30 miles to Neel Gap on the AT had me questioning whether I could really sustain that level of effort for hundreds of miles. My shoulders were killing me, and an old tendinitis injury in my knees flared up. When I hobbled into Mountain Crossings, the outfitter conveniently located right on the AT, I was more than ready to invest in lightweight gear! By swapping out my big three (shelter, sleep system, and pack) and mailing several items home, I hiked out with a 20-pound pack, feeling lighter—physically and mentally—about what lay ahead.

on trail with an article of clothing or gear item. Things that are comfortable in the store can quickly become loathed when you're sweating up a major climb. I (Heather) have dealt with more blisters than I care to admit due to shoes and boots that fit well in the store but became painfully small as soon as I was carrying a full pack and trail pronation set in!

Especially if you're new to backpacking, or if you're using a new item for the first time, it's best to test your gear before your trip. Do this in a low-stakes environment, such as your backyard or a local park. Take a few shakeout hikes, where you mimic expected trip conditions as closely as possible. Pack all the items you plan to carry on your trip. Practice packing your pack. Get used to adjusting it and carrying it with a load. Pay attention to how it feels and if there are any irritating spots. Even if you're a seasoned backpacker, whenever possible, test new gear before using it in the field.

Unfortunately, advance testing isn't always feasible, and for that reason we cover the major considerations below. How much importance to place on any one of these factors is an individual decision. Simply because an item is the lightest, most expensive, or most popular, doesn't mean it's right for you. Furthermore, bear in mind that your kit will evolve as gear wears out and items need to be replaced. At that time, you can reevaluate and make changes. For me (Katie), this understanding took a lot of pressure out of finding the "perfect" pieces of gear initially.

For recommendations, see our sample gear lists at the end of this chapter and Additional Resources.

Weight

Although weight is first in our list of factors, that doesn't mean it is of the utmost importance. However, for any long-distance backpacker, the weight you carry will become increasingly important the longer you carry it. Thus, it's within this community that the "ultralight" movement originated. Ultralight base weights are classically defined as under 10 pounds.

The term *base weight* refers to the weight of everything you carry that doesn't change in weight over the duration of your trip. This includes your empty backpack, sleeping bag, clothing, electronics, water bottles, etc. Water, fuel for your stove, and fuel for your body are not included. *Pack weight* is the sum of both the base weight and the consumables. Your pack weight will fluctuate hourly on the trail!

Obviously, there are techniques to keep the weight of your consumables lower (eating dried food, not using a stove, carrying only the water you need for that stretch of trail, etc.), and these options do not directly influence gear choices (aside from your food-preparation system and pack capacity). However, the place to invest most of your effort in weight savings is in your base weight.

The weight of each item in your pack adds up, resulting in an overall greater pack weight and additional strain on the body. By going lighter on big items like your shelter, sleeping bag, and pack (known as the "big three"), weight savings

accumulate quickly. As you gain experience and replace worn items over time, you can save additional ounces on smaller supporting items. These savings may be more modest, but they still contribute to an overall reduction in base weight.

Quality and Durability

When you're long-distance hiking, quality gear is very important. The longer your hike, the more days you are out, the more wear and tear you put on your gear. There is a reason that many companies do not offer lifetime warranties to thru-hikers! In one season, you may place the anticipated lifetime wear of an average consumer onto your gear. For this reason, you'll want to choose high-quality, durable items, with a few exceptions.

Certain items will wear out over the course of several months of hiking no matter how durable they are. These include socks, shoes, and your day-to-day hiking clothes. Other items, if chosen well, will last for years—even if you thru-hike multiple times. These include shelters, backpacks, sleeping bags, and stoves. For this reason, we encourage you to invest in quality,

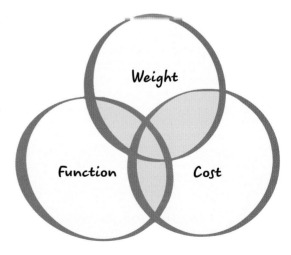

Select the gear item that most neatly fits into the overlap.

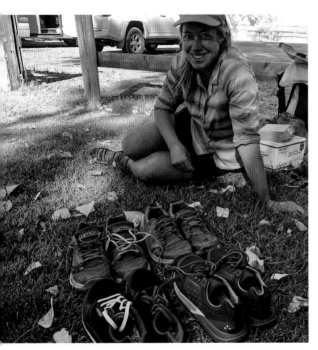

Expect to go through several pairs of shoes on a long distance hike!

prolonging time to fatigue. But they are not chosen for their durability. Most shoe companies design their shoes to last the average person 300 to 500 miles, depending on weight and frequency of use. If you choose trail-running shoes for a multi-month hike, keep in mind that you will need four to five pairs (maybe more). The heavier you are (with pack on) and the more off-trail travel you do, the faster they will wear out. This is definitely a place to search for sales to save some money.

When selecting shoes, it's also important to keep in mind that your feet will grow during a hike! Your feet will expand from the long hours of walking as well as the additional weight of a pack. Choose a half to full size larger for your

durable pieces for these long-wearing items and spend less on the ones that will wear out regardless.

The most common footwear choice for long-distance hikers is trail-running shoes. These are popular due to their flexibility, responsiveness, comfort, and drying capabilities. They are also lighter than traditional backpacking boots, requiring less energy expenditure and

Katie Tip

Extend the life of your gear by caring for it properly. At the end of each season, clean all your gear according to manufacturer instructions. Removing dirt and body oils prevents gear from wearing out as quickly. Store gear in a clean, dry area. For down items, ensure that they are kept in a way that doesn't compress the feathers, which can destroy their ability to insulate.

Heather Tip

In 2005, I was on the PCT on my second thru-hike. At that time many hikers were influenced by the only hiker-sourced guidebook and an online forum. As a result, there was what was often referred to as the PCT uniform: a Marmot PreCip jacket, Montrail Hardrock shoes, a Tarptent, and ULA backpack. While my partner and I carried a Tarptent, I had none of those other items. In group photos and any time we hung out with other hikers, I felt left out and somehow like I wasn't a "real" hiker because I wasn't carrying the "right" gear. ● Later, I received a PreCip jacket and ULA backpack as gifts. After hiking thousands of miles with those items, it finally dawned on me: neither of them worked for me. In the case of the backpack, it downright hurt me. On my second PCT thru-hike in 2013, when I set the self-supported FKT, the pack wore enormous sores on my body. It took months for them to heal after I finished my hike. Only after that experience did I get rid of it and go back to the backpack that worked for me in 2005—a Gossamer Gear backpack. ● Plenty of people use Marmot PreCip jackets and ULA packs successfully and they are good pieces. They were not the right ones for me, however.

Katie Tip

On one of my long-distance hikes, I started with a pack with which I'd already logged thousands of miles. A week into the hike, I was offered a new pack by a different manufacturer. Excited by the idea of trying something new from a reputable company, I took the opportunity. When I tried it on, it felt comfortable enough, so I loaded it up and took off for a five-day stretch, sending my original pack home. Within a few hours of hiking, the pressure of the pack on my tailbone was so uncomfortable that I held my hands underneath my lower back to keep the weight off. When I removed the pack to sit, my tailbone ached. By the time I got to my next resupply point, the damage had been done. My tailbone was bruised, causing me to change my gait, which resulted in the most painful blisters I've ever experienced. Further, the pain lingered for two months after the hike ended. It was a high-quality pack, but it wasn't the right pack for me. Lesson learned!

first pair to allow your feet to expand during the adaptation phase without blistering. Some hikers' feet never return to their previous size. For this reason, we don't recommend purchasing all of your shoes in advance of a hike, especially if it's your first long-distance trek. Additional shoes can be ordered online and shipped to your resupply points along the way.

In the same way, you don't need to spend a lot of money on performance clothing for daily wear. Hiking clothes—as opposed to insulating or shell layers—are usually the dirtiest, stinkiest, and most likely to have holes at the end of the trip, regardless of their quality. We both have used thrifted items as our everyday hiking wear to save money on these items that are usually destroyed completely after one season of heavy use. We then funnel the majority of our clothing budgets into items that we expect to carry on multiple trips, which are primarily our insulating and shell layers—the ones important for survival.

Cost

The price tag for gear and outdoor apparel can be shocking. As with many things, you get what you pay for in terms of quality, durability, functionality, and weight. This is why it's so important to determine what type of gear you need based on the factors discussed earlier in this chapter. When you get into quality backpacking gear, often the difference you pay for is a few ounces of weight, rather than significant performance differences. While a tent under 1 pound exists, ask yourself if it is worth the cost difference versus a tent that weighs 20 ounces and costs a lot less. This is the type of question only you can answer based on your unique needs and preferences. Determine which items need to be optimally functional and funnel a larger proportion of your budget into those to make the dollars stretch.

Because of the high cost, we highly recommend borrowing gear prior to purchase if possible. This can help you test and rule out items before you've spent a lot of money. There are also multiple vetting websites, such as Treeline Review, that can help you narrow your choices, and many options to purchase items used. Another cost-saving strategy is to look for previous year models and sales. Most manufacturers make only slight changes to items such as shoes, backpacks, and apparel from year to year. Sometimes the change is as small as a different color! This often means the previous year's model can be picked up at a steep discount (see Additional Resources for suggested retailer and review websites).

In the end, purchasing gear that works for you that you will use for years to come on most if not all trips is the best way to save money. Many people purchase items based on erroneous factors and end up repurchasing many gear items when they realize what it is they really like/need/want. Over time you can build an excellent kit on a budget by making wise

PERFORMANCE FABRICS STRENGTHS AND WEAKNESSES

	POLYESTER	RAYON	NYLON	SPANDEX	WOOL/ ALPACA	SILK	BAMBOO	LYOCELL	DOWN
FIBER TYPE	synthetic	manu-factured cellulose	synthetic	synthetic	protein	protein	manu-factured cellulose	manu-factured cellulose	protein
WICKING	●	●	●	●	●	●	●	●	
INSULATING OR THERMO-REGULATING	●				●				●
FAST-DRYING	●		●		● *(depending on weight)*	● *(depending on weight)*			
ANTI-ODOR			●		●	●			

choices, taking care of your gear to make it last, and paying more for the crux items and less for the supporting roles.

Functionality and Fit

Always evaluate your gear and clothing choices on personal performance. If they work for you and you don't need to change them, then don't! But if a piece doesn't fit you correctly or function the way you need it to, no matter the quality, it is the wrong piece *for you*. Avoid the mistake of thinking that you'll adapt to an item in the field or that a slightly misfitting piece is "no big deal." Over the course of hundreds of miles and thousands of footsteps, minor discomfort compounds into debilitating issues that can force you off trail. This is further exacerbated by environmental conditions such as excess heat, cold, or wetness.

When shopping for new items or borrowing gear for your trip, do not dismiss the importance of measuring yourself, trying on items, and testing them to ensure a good fit. It's particularly important to do this for your pack and footwear because in these categories, poor-fitting items can dramatically affect your comfort. For packs, follow the manufacturer's instructions on their website to determine your correct size. Don't guess! With any new-to-you pack, load it up and try it on. Adjust it and walk around in it. If there are any areas that rub uncomfortably, it's not the pack for you. Similarly, footwear is a highly personal choice. It's helpful to try on multiple pairs while wearing your favorite hiking socks. Walk around in them to ensure there are no pressure points.

Katie Tip

Thinking of your clothing as a layering system can be the key to greater comfort, safety, and a lighter pack. Your layering system may change slightly depending on the conditions of your route, but at the foundation, you have a base layer, an insulating layer, and a protective layer. The base layer wicks moisture off your skin and can include your undergarments, thermal top and bottom, and hiking clothes. The insulating layer retains body heat and includes items like a fleece top or down jacket. The protective layer shields you from the elements and includes a rain jacket and pants. You can adjust to varying weather conditions and regulate body temperature by adding or removing layers. Avoid excess pack weight by removing redundant items.

Fabric

The most important functions of fabric in outdoor apparel and gear are simple: wicking, fast-drying, waterproof, and insulating. Depending on what item you are examining, the optimal properties are likely a combination of these. Staying warm and dry is the key to happiness and survival in the backcountry!

Most backpacks, tents, and shells rely on some form of nylon or Dyneema Composite Fabric. These versatile fabrics have varying capacities for waterproofness, durability, and drying speed based on their thickness, weave, cut, and/or topical treatments. Your choice of fabrics in these cases will usually come down to cost and weight.

When it comes to hiking apparel, there are a wide range of popularly used fabrics. Polyester and spandex are the most common synthetics, while merino wool is the most commonly used natural fabric. Within one item, fibers can be mixed to add different properties, such as nylon for durability and spandex for stretch. See the Performance Fabrics Table for a comparison of strengths and weaknesses.

If you haven't heard it yet, you likely will . . . in the backcountry "cotton kills!" This statement is a bit dramatic, considering that for many years people backpacked in denim shorts and cotton T-shirts! But cotton does the exact opposite of those important functions mentioned earlier—it is slow to dry, non-insulative, and not at all water resistant. Wearing items made from cotton increases your likelihood of chafing and discomfort, as well as your risk of hypothermia in cold, wet conditions. Not all cellulose fabrics are created equal, though, and some, such as linen, bamboo, or lyocell, are even appropriate in certain conditions.

Used versus New

As noted, outfitting yourself with the necessary gear can be expensive. This is compounded every time you purchase an item that doesn't

Heather Tip

A note on natural versus synthetic fabrics: In 2003, I thru-hiked the AT wearing mostly cotton-poly blends from a discount store. These were an upgrade from the selection of cotton T-shirts taken from my closet at home that I'd started with! However, after four months of soggy, stinky clothing, I was elated to discover a new trend in the activewear market: merino wool. ● I saved up to purchase a merino base layer set from Icebreaker, and it was my prized possession on the PCT in 2005 and the CDT in 2006. Those layers were comfortable, kept me warm when they got wet, and—best of all—did not stink. Fast-forward many years, and I have found multiple reasons to wear natural fabrics on trail. The lack of odor after days of wear is one of them. Another is my decision to move away from synthetic clothing, which is made from fossil fuels. ● Another benefit to choosing natural fabrics: a reduction in microplastic pollution. Microplastics are tiny particles (smaller than 5 mm) that are shed by synthetic fabrics. It is estimated that a single fleece can shed hundreds of thousands of these in a lifetime of use. Since plastics take hundreds of years to decompose, they have become bioaccumulative in our environment—primarily our waterways but also in plant, animal, and human tissues. ● Numerous companies produce merino activewear now, and there are even companies such as Appalachian Gear Company that have branched into alpaca wear. Lyocell (made from trees) and bamboo fabrics, when made in low-pollution manners, are also burgeoning industries in nonpetroleum-based activewear textiles.

work for you and you have to buy something else. For this reason, we recommend keeping your initial investment low by trying before you buy—either by borrowing from friends or through rental programs—this allows you to take things for a test hike rather than just trying it on in a store or selecting it from an online source. Look for local outdoors clubs that may have loaner gear for you to try out.

If you decide to go this route, make sure borrowed gear fits you properly! At best, poorly fitting gear can be annoying. At worst, it can result in injury and a premature end to your trip. Because good fit is critical for certain items such as footwear, it's recommended that you purchase those new. A well-fitting pack is also essential, so take extra care to ensure good fit when borrowing one.

When previewing an item isn't possible, a way to save money is to purchase used. There are many online sites that cater to this market. These range from mega-sites like eBay to niche Facebook groups. The most important thing to do when purchasing used gear online is to know your source as well as what protections you have from the hosting website if items are being bought and sold through third parties.

Another option is to seek out used gear stores near you. Some outdoor retailers have regular used gear sales called Garage Sales. These can be excellent places to find flawed items that are still serviceable. REI also stocks many of these items online year-round as well. Other options include your standard thrift stores as well as independent gear stores. It's often preferable to shop in person because you can gauge the wear and tear on the item yourself, rather than relying on another person's evaluation.

Although used items may not serve you as long as their new counterparts would, buying used offers an opportunity to try things out at a discounted price before committing to spending the money on brand-new. Many items, if gently used, may give you years of functionality for a fraction of the cost. You can build out your kit with a combination of used and new gear and upgrade piece by piece as items wear out. See Additional Resources for a list of used gear websites.

PRIMARY GEAR

In this section we discuss the major types of gear: the big three plus food preparation. This

Katie Tip

Simulate a frame in a frameless pack by using a folded sleeping pad inside the pack on the portion that goes against your back. This adds structure to the pack and prevents objects from pressing into your back, creating more comfort overall.

quadfecta of gear items forms the core of your kit and has the most impact on your comfort (aside from footwear) and survival.

Packs

Your pack has one job: to carry your gear. Yet its fit and function are paramount to your comfort on the trail—and comfort is very closely entwined with success. A poorly fitting pack will make you miserable, and since you will be wearing your pack all day every day, it has the potential to ruin your trip if it doesn't fit well. For that reason, packs (along with shoes) are the most personal and tricky gear items to purchase without trying them out first.

The capacity of the pack you need is dictated by the size and weight of your gear as well as how much additional space you need to accommodate your food and water (determined, in part, by how frequent your resupply will be). Therefore, we recommend purchasing this item after you have a sense of the other gear you'll be carrying. Once you know the load-carrying capacity you need, you can evaluate the pack's weight and additional features, like pockets and fabrics. Here, we discuss two basic types of packs to get you started in your research.

Packs with Frames

For decades, packs with frames have been the standard for recreational backpacking. Mid-twentieth-century packs used external frames with frame bags hung on them. In the latter part of the century, internal frame packs were developed. In these the frames are completely hidden. The internal frame pack is the primary framed backpack seen on trail these days and the one we focus on here.

The benefit of a framed pack is its load distribution. The rigid frame is anchored between the shoulder straps and hip belt, transferring the weight of the pack off your shoulders and onto your hips. Since the pelvis is anatomically designed to be weight bearing, framed packs use natural bone structure to carry loads efficiently.

Framed packs become more beneficial the heavier your pack weight becomes. Most people find that pack weights of more than 25 pounds are uncomfortable without a frame and hip belt to transfer the load. Framed packs can have metal, plastic, or carbon-fiber frames and weigh

Large boulders serve as a windbreak in an alpine camp.

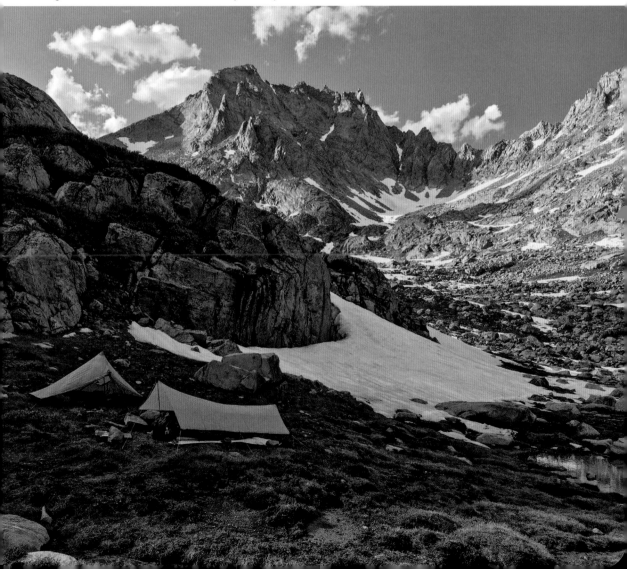

from just over 1 pound to upwards of almost 10 pounds empty. When choosing a pack, keep in mind that the weight of the pack itself counts toward your base weight. Heavier framed packs often have more padding and better weight distribution, but you'll carry that suspension system no matter how light the rest of your load is.

Frameless Packs

Frameless packs, on the other hand, are best suited for lighter pack weights. The packs themselves are very light, sometimes less than a pound, since they do not include the weight of a frame. They are usually simple in design and are comparable to the rucksacks used before framed packs became commonplace. Frameless packs are very popular on long-distance trails because of their weight savings. However, most frameless packs have a load rating that needs to be heeded both for the durability of the backpack and for the comfort of the hiker. Without a frame and because of the lighter-weight materials used to keep these packs minimal, they are not as well-suited to carrying heavy loads, and the lack of structure causes more of the weight to hang on the shoulders. Therefore, chronic overloading of a frameless pack will lead to bodily discomfort and likely to pack failure.

When choosing between a framed and frameless pack, be honest about the weight load you will be carrying the majority of the time—not outlier days—and choose according to manufacturer specs. Take into consideration your total weight (not base weight) during your longest food or water carries—that is, your longest stretch between resupply and/or water sources—and how often carries of that length will occur on a given trip. Saving a few ounces by opting for a frameless pack can be catastrophic on a long-distance trail when your shoulder strap comes completely unstitched due to chronic overloading a hundred miles from the nearest road! When evaluating a pack, keep in mind the additional features that can affect the load-carrying capacity, including compression straps, hip and shoulder straps, load lifter straps, and a sternum strap.

Shelters

The place you call home each night on the trail is not only a critical piece of gear; it can serve as an anchor of continuity in the midst of an ever-changing journey. At the very least, your shelter needs to be adequate to protect you from the elements expected on your particular hike. Ideally it will also be easy to set up in a variety of conditions and durable enough to last for many years. There are several types of shelter systems; here, we discuss those that are most popular among long-distance hikers.

Tarps

The tarp is the most basic of shelters and is often the lightest, though due to the increasing availability of ultralight materials this is not always the case. Tarps are usually simple rectangles (although some do have some aerodynamic shaping) made from waterproof fabric with anchor points in various places so that they can be tied out to trees, rocks, bushes, or any other solid object. Often, trekking poles are used to create structure. In order to function well, they must cover a fairly large area, although you can position your sleeping pad in any configuration that works underneath. For this reason, tarps are popular in areas where there are no established campsites.

Tarps offer a wide degree of versatility and can be adapted to weather conditions through versatile pitching configurations, use of natural weather blocks, and modular components, such as bug netting and flooring. And with open-ended pitches, (meaning the ends are open so that air can flow through), they also offer supreme ventilation, reducing the likelihood of condensation.

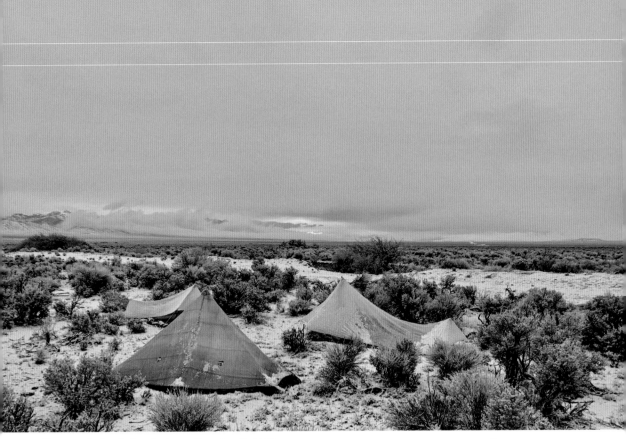

Choose a shelter that protects you from the elements.

Although tarps are simplistic, the learning curve for setting them up well in inclement weather is rather steep. You also must be able to locate the correct number and type of natural anchors. This can be challenging in desert areas and other treeless areas. Most tarp users are quite devoted to their systems once they've mastered pitching them in creative ways.

Tents

The tent is by far the most popular shelter in the backcountry. They tend to be more intuitive in their setup and offer more environmental protection than tarps. Tents range in style, size, and design from 1-pound single-person summer tents to enormous multi-person four-season tents. Tents are the piece of gear with the most wide-ranging component materials for weight,

durability, and season. Because of this, no matter what you are looking for in a shelter, there is a tent that meets your needs.

Single-Walled Tents

The majority of long-distance hikers using tents will choose a single-walled design. These tents are the lightest option and are composed of a waterproof fabric upper and bug netting sides. The floors are sometimes the same as the upper or they may be untreated nylon. These tents are often designed to be set up with trekking poles in order to further reduce the amount of weight that needs to be carried.

The primary benefits of using a single-walled tent are their lighter weight, simple setup, and small footprint. Drawbacks include condensation issues and a moderate learning curve in

53

the pitch in order to establish proper tension. Single-walled tents range in design from glorified tarps to hybrid poncho tents to complex freestanding tents with multiple vestibules and entrances.

Double-Walled Tents

Double-walled tents differ from single-walled in that the tent itself is usually nylon and netting and is not waterproof. A separate rain fly made from waterproof materials is clipped on over the top of the main tent when inclement weather is anticipated. Double-walled tents are typically quite heavy due to the weight of two separate tent layers and poles, but as demand for lighter options continues, manufacturers are producing lighter three-season versions that are popular among long-distance hikers.

The primary benefits to choosing a double-walled tent are versatility in airflow, fewer issues with condensation, and ease of setup with proprietary poles. The main drawback is the weight.

Hammocks

Hammocks have become increasingly popular in recent years. Like tarps, they require natural anchor points to set them up. This makes them best suited for forested trails. However, creative and experienced hammock users successfully

set them up everywhere they hike—even desert landscapes!

The primary advantages of hammocks is that, unlike a tarp or tent, they do not rely on cleared areas to camp. This makes them an excellent option for areas with lush understories, such as East Coast trails like the AT. The limitations include the lack of internal or vestibular space for gear, heat loss without additional gear such as an under quilt, and the steep learning curve for proper setup, especially in areas with fewer natural anchors. Use of natural anchors may be restricted in some areas to protect the local flora and other features, so research the viability of using a hammock before leaving home. Hammocks may also be on the heavier side due to the material needed to support body weight.

Sleeping Systems

While not quite as varied as shelters, there are a few options for sleep systems, and it largely comes down to preference. Certain types of sleepers (side vs. back, cold vs. warm) will find specific combinations more practical for them. The sleep system is made up of a pad to insulate from heat loss to the ground and an insulating cover. In this section, we cover two types from each category: solid and inflatable pads, and sleeping bags and quilts.

Solid Pads

Solid sleeping pads are typically made of a closed-cell foam. These come in a variety of thicknesses and lengths as well as channel or egg-crate designs. The composition of different pads impacts their durability and insulative properties. A pad's R-value measures its insulative properties: the higher the R-value, the warmer the pad will keep you. In general, any pad that does not list an R-value is not a good choice for the backcountry. Many long-distance hikers carry pads that measure 3 for three-season hiking; R-values of at least 5

THE SEVEN PRINCIPLES OF LEAVE NO TRACE

1. Plan Ahead and Prepare
2. Travel and Camp on Durable Surfaces
3. Dispose of Waste Properly
4. Leave What You Find
5. Minimize Campfire Impacts
6. Respect Wildlife
7. Be Considerate of Other Visitors

are necessary for snow/winter-weather camping. Design features such as channeling or egg-crate molded foam are meant to increase R-value.

The main benefit of a solid pad is that they are nearly indestructible when it comes to punctures and tears. Additionally, they are inexpensive and easily modifiable (e.g., cutting off sections to create a torso-length pad, which saves on weight). The main drawback is that they are bulky, but because of their durability, they can be carried on the outside of a backpack without fear of damage, unlike an inflatable pad. Solid pads are also thinner, meaning you'll feel the ground through them, but this also usually makes them the lightest option.

Inflatable Pads

Inflatable pads are typically regarded as the most comfortable backcountry pad. They vary widely in styles and R-values. Some are self-inflating (although you will need to blow them up partially) and others require total manual inflation. Depending on the interior insulation used to create R-value, some are very crinkly when you move around on them. This can be annoying to your tent mates . . . or other people camped nearby!

The main advantages of inflatable pads are their comfort and compactness. They can also be stacked on top of a solid pad to increase insulative properties since R-value is cumulative. Their main drawback is that they are susceptible to punctures, leaks, and tears. Carrying a patch kit is a must, and successfully stopping leaks is not always a guarantee. Inflatable pads also tend to be more expensive than foam pads.

Sleeping Bags

Sleeping bags are the main insulative cover that most people think of when they think of camping. They work by trapping body-warmed air and reducing convective heat loss. They come in synthetic and down versions, with down being the best warmth-to-weight ratio. Synthetic bags are typically less expensive and retain their insulating properties even if they get wet (though conductive heat loss would occur in a wet bag). Down must be kept dry in order for it to perform optimally. In 2014, water-resistant down became available, enabling down to retain its loft better when wet and to dry faster than conventional down.

Sleeping bags can have a variety of cuts, lengths, and warmth ratings. Finding one that fits you well without a lot of excess air space to heat is the key to getting the best performance from your bag. If you are a smaller person, look for petite or women's-specific models in order to ensure good fit.

Warmth ratings are not always accurate. While there are international standards—ISO or EN (International Standards Organization or European Norm, respectively)—not all companies use these. To further complicate matters, these standardized ratings calculate multiple warmth ratings for each bag! Why? To give a better scope of the overall performance of the bag itself. Each bag will have a comfort rating (where a colder sleeper will be comfortable), a lower-limit rating at which a warm sleeper will be comfortable, and sometimes an extreme rating (where the sleeper will survive, but not be comfortable).

Due to all of these factors, companies may label a bag as 0-degree, but it may not be a 0-degree bag for you. Be sure to find out which rating the 0 actually is. If you purchase a bag with an extreme rating of 0 degrees, you'll be pretty uncomfortable if you try sleeping in it at that temperature. The same goes for whether you are a cold or warm sleeper. Women's bags are generally marketed at their comfort rating because the average woman sleeps colder than the average man. A unisex bag is likely to be marketed at the lower-limit rating.

Choosing the right warmth sleeping bag can be complicated, but once you find a good bag, it should last you many years. Take the time to research your options before you buy. In general, if you tend to be a colder sleeper, get a sleeping bag rated down to 10 degrees colder than the coldest nights you expect to be camping in.

Sleeping Quilts

Sleeping quilts are increasingly popular with ultralight hikers, couples, and long-distance hikers in general. The main reasons for this are the weight savings and the freedom of movement. Some people feel very restricted in the classic sleeping bag. A quilt, on the other hand, is essentially a comforter like you'd use on your bed at home, with either straps or a single piece of fabric on the bottom to attach to the sleeping pad, rather than insulation. Quilts also lack a hood and zippers as you would find on a traditional mummy-style sleeping bag. This makes them much lighter than a similarly rated sleeping bag due to fewer materials used in construction.

Quilts can be made from synthetic or down insulation with the same pros and cons as in

Katie's summer thru-hiking kit

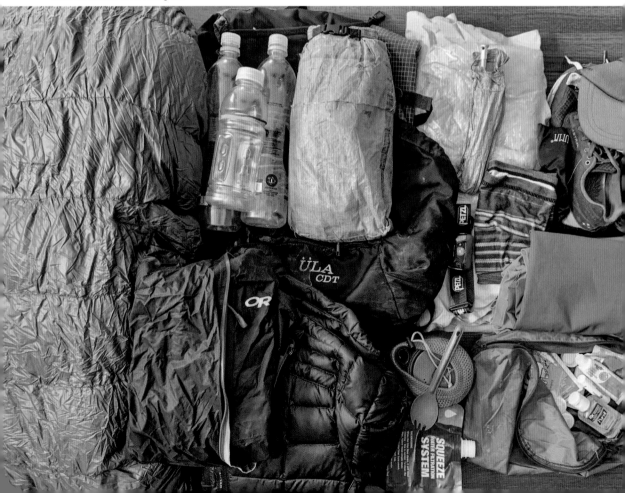

a traditional sleeping bag. They are popular choices for couples since a double quilt allows them to sleep next to one another and share body warmth. This means your quilt for two can weigh even less than a single sleeping bag, and the weight is shared between two people.

Quilts are rated similarly to sleeping bags, although not all companies will have them rated according to the international standard, so be certain to ask how their quilts are rated, just as you would for a sleeping bag. Quilts may not be a good choice for active sleepers due to the possibility they'll shift open in the night and allow drafts, although many have straps that allow you to attach the quilt to your sleeping pad, minimizing this issue.

Sleeping bags and quilts are one of those items where investing in a quality piece is recommended. Higher-end products usually have a greater warmth-to-weight ratio and are more durable. Get the best you can afford.

Food Preparation

Among long-distance hikers there are two very staunch food-preparation camps: those that cook and those that go stoveless. The choice boils down to preference and route conditions, although it may be necessary to forego a stove in some areas when there are extensive fire bans. We personally choose to go stoveless on trails like the PCT, which has a relatively dry and warm climate for the majority of the hiking season, and carry a stove in areas that are usually cooler or wetter, such as high routes or shoulder-season trips.

Preparing Food Without a Stove

Hikers who elect not to carry a stove typically eschew any stove and its accompanying fuel in order to save weight. Instead, they usually rely on foods that are ready to eat, such as bars, trail mix, and jerky, while supplementing with soaked meals. Soaking your food is exactly

Heather Tip
Testing meals at home to see how well they soak is crucial! I have definitely skipped this step and subsequently had to choke down some barely edible meals that only partially rehydrated. This led to difficulty with digestion to say the least. It's well worth the time and extra cost to prep one of each candidate meal beforehand to ensure that the soaking method works and your on-trail experience is tasty!

what it sounds like: water is added to dehydrated or freeze-dried food and allowed to sit until it's rehydrated. Although often referred to as cold-soaking or eating cold, both terms are misnomers since the food will be at ambient air temperature. *No-cook* is a more accurate name for the stoveless soak method.

The main advantage of no-cook soaking is the simplicity and weight savings as well as not having to plan for replenishing fuel along the way. The primary drawback is that some meals can take a very long time to rehydrate (if they do so at all), especially commercial dried meals intended for hot-water rehydration. If you are trying this method out, we recommend experimenting at home to determine what foods rehydrate best and to gauge how long it takes.

Preparing Food With a Stove

Stove-based food systems are essentially a warm version of soaking. Although the term *soaking* is almost exclusively used to refer to stoveless preparation, there are very few individuals who actually *cook* on trail. Typically, stove-based "cooking" simply means adding hot water to freeze-dried or dehydrated meals, or simmering quick-cook foods such as Knorr sides or ramen. Because of this, the main difference with the stove-based method is the weight of the fuel and stove.

The primary benefit of stove-based food systems is warm food. This is a comfort benefit and

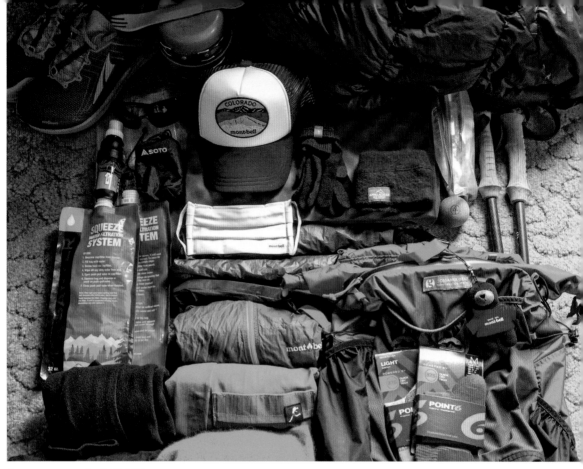

A summer gear cube for Heather

can also be a survival benefit if needed. Someone who is bordering on hypothermia will warm up much faster consuming warm liquids than shivering in a sleeping bag. The main drawback to using a stove is the weight and the need to replenish fuel along the way, which can sometimes be difficult.

It should also be noted that in some places, especially the American West, stove and campfire bans are common due to drought conditions, and special permits may be required in order to use camp stoves in the backcountry. Keeping tabs on these regulations can add another level of complexity to trip planning, especially on long trips that pass through many management areas.

TIPS FOR LIGHTWEIGHT BACKCOUNTRY TRAVEL

While there's more to gear than achieving the lightest pack weight, it's true that a lighter pack can reduce strain on your body, enable you to hike more miles comfortably, and improve the overall enjoyment of your trip. With the advances in lightweight backcountry gear in recent decades, most individuals can assemble a sub-20-pound base weight without breaking their budget and while still carrying the necessary gear to stay safe.

The first step to reducing pack weight is to weigh all of your items on an accurate scale, such as a postal scale, and track data on a spreadsheet. Remember, for the biggest impact, focus on acquiring lighter items for the big three. Maximizing multipurpose items and eliminating nonessentials, such as a mirror or deodorant, also shaves ounces. As you gain experience, you'll have a better idea of which items you actually do and do not need and which items can serve multiple purposes. In your effort to reduce pack weight, be sure to never compromise safety! There are certain items, such as a personal locator beacon (PLB), that you may never use, but which should always remain in your kit (see chapter 3 for more on PLBs).

Lightweight backcountry travel isn't solely about the physical weight of your gear. It is also about the weight of your impact on the landscape you are traversing. We recommend visiting the Leave No Trace website to learn more about the seven principles of Leave No Trace

(see Additional Resources). These principles provide an adaptable framework to maximize enjoyment for all outdoor recreationists and protect the ecosystems we visit (see "The Seven Principles of Leave No Trace" earlier sidebar).

"Katie's Summer Gear List" details the kit I (Katie) carried on a southbound hike of the CDT from June through September. This represents my standard summer setup, and I further refine it based on the specific route I'm hiking. Shoulder-season swaps and reasons for certain items are noted.

"Heather's Summer Gear List" is what I (Heather) typically carry on multi-night treks in the months of June, July, and August. Swaps and additions for shoulder-season months (May, September) are noted along with some selection reasons.

KATIE'S SUMMER GEAR LIST			
ITEM	**WEIGHT IN OZ**		**NOTES AND SHOULDER SEASON (SS) TWEAKS**
PACK	**CARRIED**	**WORN**	
ULA CDT	24		
Trash compactor bag	1.2		Waterproof liner to keep pack contents dry
FOOD SYSTEM			
TOAKS titanium alcohol stove	1.8		Includes windscreen, stand, and carrying bag
TOAKS 550-ml titanium pot with lid	2.6		
TOAKS titanium long-handled spoon	0.57		
Loksak Opsak 12" by 20"	1		Used to reduce food odors that attract animals
Granite Gear food sack	1		
SHELTER			
Zpacks Hexamid	10.4		Includes stuff sack and guylines
Polycryo ground cloth	1.5		Vapor barrier from the ground
Six Moon Designs stakes (6)	2.3		
Leki Micro Vario Carbon trekking poles	15		Use both while hiking and as poles for tent
DITTIES			
Six Moon Designs 2L pack pod	0.7		Used to store ditties
Suunto compass	1.6		
Mini pocketknife	0.6		
Contact case, contacts, glasses	3		

KATIE'S SUMMER GEAR LIST, CONTINUED			
ITEM	**WEIGHT IN OZ**		**NOTES AND SHOULDER SEASON (SS) TWEAKS**
DITTIES	**CARRIED**	**WORN**	
Toothpaste, toothbrush	1		
Hothands hand warmers (2)	1.6		
Sewing kit	0.1		
Triple antibiotic ointment	0.5		
Joshua Tree salve	0.5		For skin care
Ibuprofen, Benadryl	0.3		
Tenacious Tape	0.1		All-purpose repair tape made for gear
Mesh repair kit	0.1		For bug netting of tent
Therm-a-Rest patch kit	0.1		For sleeping pad
Leukotape	0.2		All-purpose medical tape that stays stuck
Hand sanitizer	0.5		
Moleskin	0.1		
Sawyer sunscreen	0.6		
Head net	0.1		
Tick-removal tweezers	0.4		
Extra Sawyer gasket	0.1		For water filter
Mini lighter	0.4		
Diva Cup	0.5		
Pen or magic marker	0.2		
Mini journal	2		
SLEEP			
Therm-a-Rest NeoAir small	8		I sleep with my empty pack under my legs
Katabatic Gear Sawatch (15-degree quilt, 900fp) in waterproof sack	25		Swap for ZPacks 20-degree bag in warm weather; I'm a cold sleeper
CLOTHES			
Visor		0.8	
Sunglasses		0.7	
Montbell down jacket	9		
Astral trail-running shoes		20	
Point6 extra-light mini crew hiking socks (2 pair)	1.5	1.5	
Point6 mid-calf socks	2		Only for sleeping
Purple Rain hiking dress		5.3	
Icebreaker midweight tights	6.5		
Thin long-sleeve shirt		6	Swap for fleece midlayer in SS
ExOfficio briefs		1	
Sports bra		1.5	
Outdoor Research Helium II rain jacket	5.8		
Liner gloves	1.2		Add fleece mittens for SS
Rain mitts	1.3		

KATIE'S SUMMER GEAR LIST, CONTINUED			
ITEM	**WEIGHT IN OZ**		**NOTES AND SHOULDER SEASON (SS) TWEAKS**
CLOTHES	**CARRIED**	**WORN**	
ZPacks fleece beanie	1		Add balaclava in cold weather
Buff	1		
HYDRATION			
Sawyer Squeeze Filter and backflush syringe	4		
Smartwater 1L bottle (2)	2.6		Add collapsible pouches in arid environments
ELECTRONICS			
Smartphone	10		With LifeProof case and charger cord
Anker 10,000 mAh external battery	6.4		With charger cord
Nitecore NU25 headlamp	1.2		With charger cord
Garmin inReach Mini	3.5		With charger cord
GUIDES			
Maps	varies		
Cal Topo, Gaia GPS	0		Phone apps
WALLET			
ID and credit card	1		Stored inside a ziplock bag
TOTAL CARRIED	**167.67**		
TOTAL WORN		**36.8**	

HEATHER'S SUMMER GEAR LIST			
ITEM	**WEIGHT IN OZ**		**NOTES AND SHOULDER SEASON (SS) TWEAKS**
PACK	**CARRIED**	**WORN**	
Gossamer Gear Gorilla 50 L backpack	25		Gossamer Gear Mariposa size small w/small hip belt used in SS or with heavy/bulky loads
Gossamer Gear shoulder pockets (2 large)	2.8		
Trash compactor bag	1.2		Waterproof liner to keep pack contents dry
Gossamer Gear stuff sacks	2		Used to organize clothing and food inside the pack
FOOD SYSTEM			
Humangear GoBites Duo	0.8		
Loksak Opsaks	5		Used to reduce odors that attract animals
Soto WindMaster stove	2.3		
Titanium pot	4		
SHELTER			
Gossamer Gear The One	22.4		Gossamer Gear The Two for hiking with a partner
Gossamer Gear Polycryo ground cloth	1.6		Vapor barrier from the ground
Gossamer Gear LT5 trekking poles	4.6		Use both while hiking and as poles for tent

ITEM	WEIGHT IN OZ		NOTES AND SHOULDER SEASON (SS) TWEAKS
HEATHER'S SUMMER GEAR LIST, CONTINUED			
	CARRIED	**WORN**	
DITTIES			
Rawlogy mini cork massage ball	0.7		Self-care tool
Compass	1.75		
Chamois Butt'r individual	1		Chafe prevention
Swiss Army classic knife	0.8		Knife and scissors
Toothpaste, toothbrush	1.3		
Hothands hand warmers (2)	1.7		
Sewing kit	0.1		
Neosporin	0.5		
Imodium, Benadryl, Aleve	0.3		
Pepto Bismol tablets	0.3		
Tenacious Tape	0.1		All-purpose repair tape made for gear
Mesh repair kit	0.1		For bug netting of tent
Floss sticks	0.3		
Leukotape	0.2		All-purpose medical tape that stays stuck
Hand sanitizer	0.5		
Wet wipes	3		
Sawyer Blist-O-Ban	0.1		
Sawyer sunscreen	0.6		
Sawyer Picaridin insect repellent	0.3		Remove from pack for SS
Eyedrops and extra contact lenses	0.6		
Lambswool	0.2		Excellent for between-toe blisters
Bear bagging rope	1.5		
Tick-removal tweezers	0.4		
Mask-IT feminine hygiene odor-proof disposal bags	0.5		
SLEEP			
Cuddleduds fleece pants	4.7		Add Montbell down booties for SS
Cuddleduds fleece shirt	3.7		
Point6 compression socks	2.6		Switch to thicker and nonrestrictive socks for SS
Thinlight Foam Pad	2.4		
Montbell UL Comfort System pillow	2.1		
Nightlight torso-length sleeping pad	3.4		Swap for Montbell Alpine pad (self-inflating) for SS
Montbell Down Hugger 900 #2 (34-degree comfort) sleeping bag	24		Add an Appalachian Gear Company alpaca liner for SS
Outdoor Research waterproof bag	1.4		Switch to larger size as needed in SS

HEATHER'S SUMMER GEAR LIST, CONTINUED			
ITEM	**WEIGHT IN OZ**		**NOTES AND SHOULDER SEASON (SS) TWEAKS**
CLOTHES	**CARRIED**	**WORN**	
Trucker hat		2	
Sunglasses		1.2	
Bandana	0.5		
Outdoor Research sun gloves		0.7	Swap for double fleece mittens in SS
Fleece gloves	1		Swap for wool liner in SS
Merino tank or short sleeve		4	Swap for thin long-sleeve wool top in SS
Ibex Balance briefs		1.7	
Montbell UL Thermawrap jacket	7		Add Appalachian Gear Company alpaca hoodie and Montbell Plasma 1000 jacket for SS
Altra Lone Peak trail-running shoes		25	
Point6 extra-light mini crew hiking socks (2 pair)	1.5	1.5	
Montbell Wickron stretch trail skirt		2.8	Add thin wool tights for SS
Ibex Balance bra		1.7	
Montbell Versalite rain jacket	6		
Altra trail gaiters		1.6	
Montbell Versalite pants	3		
Appalachian Gear Company beanie	1		Alpaca hat warm when wet
HYDRATION			
Sawyer All in One filter and backflush syringe	4		
MiiR reusable stainless-steel bottle	2.5		Add thermos for SS
Sawyer 64-oz pouches (2)	2.8		
ELECTRONICS			
Smartphone	10		With charger cord
External rechargable phone charger	6.5		
Outdoor Research Sensor Dry envelope	1		Store and protect electronics from rain
Black Diamond Storm headlamp	2.9		
Extra batteries	3		
Multi USB wall charger	3		
GUIDES			
Maps	varies		
Farout app	0		Where applicable. Alternatively I use Gaia GPS.
TOTAL CARRIED	**188.55**		
TOTAL WORN		**42.2**	

3
BACKCOUNTRY SAFETY

BY *Heather*

Aren't you afraid of bears?"
This is one of the most common questions I receive as a backpacker. And yet, as you'll discover in this chapter, animals (bears or otherwise) are relatively low on the backcountry risk-factor list. Why, then, does everyone ask about them? Likely because when animal attacks do occur, they are sensationalized and feed our primal fears. But most backcountry-safety concerns fall into other categories.

Backpacking is a fairly safe hobby. In fact, being out on trails is generally safer than the streets of a major city. You can of course make it more "epic" by certain choices you make. The goal of this chapter is to inform you of potential risks in several broad categories as well as provide some mitigation practices so that you can learn how to evaluate potential risks on your own routes and consider and develop action plans for different situations. This is by no means comprehensive, nor is it an assurance that nothing danger-ous will ever happen to you if you plan ahead. However, learning to evaluate risk in your unique situations and using forethought can go a long way toward keeping you safer.

The broad categories of risk covered in this chapter are weather, physical preparedness and injury, human interaction, animal interaction, water and snow, and solo hiking. Each of these categories is vast, and only a few scenarios for each will be covered. These should prime you to continue conducting specific-route risk assessments on your own. The one major category of risk and safety not covered in this chapter is navigation and route preparedness: we've devoted the entirety of chapter 4 to this topic because your ability to navigate in the backcountry is essential to your safety and enjoyment.

At the end of this book is an Assessing Risk Checklist that you may use to evaluate risk factors for specific routes. We have also included an Itinerary & Emergency Contact Worksheet that you may replicate and leave with a trusted individual.

WEATHER-RELATED RISKS

The most dangerous force in the outdoors is the weather, so protecting yourself from the negative and potentially dangerous impacts of weather and climate is the most important thing you can do.

I grew up in Michigan and learned to hike at the Grand Canyon, where I had a summer job at the South Rim of the national park when I was twenty years old. Unbeknownst to me at the time, summer is not prime hiking season in Arizona! I made many mistakes with regard to water and hiking in the heat of the day. One day I even headed out to hike along the exposed Rim Trail during a thunderstorm with lightning striking dangerously close. Years later, as an experienced backpacker, I can only shake my head and be thankful that I survived my learning curve!

Katie Tip

The scariest moments I've experienced in the backcountry have been linked to inclement weather. I've been caught in whiteout blizzard conditions without proper gear, my hands have become unusable in freezing rain, and I've nearly been hit by lightning, to name a few. Looking back, the danger in those situations could have been reduced with better research and preparation. ● Some weather concerns are unexpected and unavoidable, but you can often prepare for—or at least mitigate the risks of—many conditions. Learn to read backcountry weather and how to properly research conditions before your trip (this book can help!). Understanding the climate and general weather patterns of an area before you travel there is important, as is checking the forecast a few days before embarking on your trip. Don't underestimate the power of the weather. It can change rapidly and can turn a pleasant day into a life-threatening outing.

Backpacking versus Day Hiking

Compared to day hiking, backpacking increases weather-related risks because you will be staying out over multiple nights. Day hiking ends at a car (or building), where you can turn on the heat or air conditioning and be showered and fed within a short time. But when backpacking, factors such as nighttime temperature drops, wind, and precipitation will affect your planning and preparation as well as your actions on trail when camping out. Even in the desert, where you can see triple-digit temperatures in the day, overnight temps can often plummet dozens of degrees. Staying out overnight means having the correct sleeping bag, tent, and campsite to stay safe from the elements.

Clothing layers are always important when in the backcountry, and they become even more crucial when you're out overnight. Be diligent about adding and removing layers throughout the day to ensure your temperature and sweat rate are regulated while moving. You'll want to ensure your sleeping bag always stays dry, and I also recommend keeping a set of layers to sleep in that stay dry as well. In an emergency, having dry clothes and a dry bag can save your life.

Finding a safe campsite takes practice and attentiveness. Make a good choice by paying attention to your surroundings: Avoid camping under dead trees or limbs, especially suspended ones that could fall on you in the night. Learn some basic meteorological principles, such as what different types of clouds indicate, and be willing to revise your hiking plan according to your observations. If you see a storm building, it can be worth setting up camp early if the terrain dictates it.

Climate and Altitude

My experiences in Arizona are an extreme example since the state has many different climates and weather patterns, but no matter where you are, you can't escape the weather. Patterns of weather in certain areas form what we call climate, and the type of climate you hike in is often impacted by altitude. Understanding these complex relationships at a basic level is key to staying safe from weather-related risks when you're backpacking.

If you hike in the region you live in, you're likely already familiar with the climate. However, if your route takes you to another area altogether (or a familiar area at a different season), you'll need to do some research. The most important step before any trip is to find out the weather forecast for the period of time you will be out. You can use any number of resources for this, but I recommend NOAA weather for destinations in the United States. Use their point-and-click map, rather than a nearby zip code, in order to obtain the forecast for where you're actually going as hiking trails are generally much higher in elevation than any nearby towns, and the forecast could be drastically different for your destination.

Many complex meteorological factors create different climates at varying altitudes, even if

CAMPSITE RISK INDICATORS

- Snagged dead branches or trees over tent
- Exposed terrain or above tree line
- Open to strong prevailing winds
- Evidence of animals (scat, tracks, digs, etc.)
- Trash, broken glass, etc.
- Wet or depressed landscape in rainy weather

those areas are near one another geographically. In-depth treatment of these factors is outside the scope of this book. Generally speaking—in the Northern Hemisphere—moving upward in elevation results in climatic shifts equivalent to moving northward. This is why the very high mountains around places like Tucson, Arizona, have pine trees and snowfall when the desert below is hot and dry. It's imperative to get the forecast for the altitude you'll be backpacking in, rather than simply a nearby locale, which may be at a different elevation.

Once you have your forecast, use that information to pack appropriately. Be sure to carry adequate raingear, a proper shelter, a correctly rated sleeping bag and sleeping pad, etc. In addition to the forecast for your trip, reference the climate data for the region. Knowing the broader weather potential for where you are headed can help you make decisions that cover worst-case scenarios if the forecast changes while you're out there. This is especially important for longer trips and for trips that require a long travel period beforehand. Your forecast from home may be dry and warm, but if the weather patterns and averages indicate that rain and cooler nights are typical for the time of year you will be there, err on the side of caution and pack for the average. Forecasts are often only reliable twelve to twenty-four hours out and are often less accurate in mountainous regions due to the complexity of meteorological factors at play.

Lightning

Perhaps the most dramatic weather risk of all is lightning. It can be a serious risk anytime you are hiking during a storm but especially when you are above tree line. The best place to be during a storm that includes lightning is inside of a building, but of course that is not possible when you're backpacking. I have been caught above tree line in lightning many times in my hiking and backpacking experiences, and running for cover from the storms will always remain among my most vivid memories from any hike. Certain areas, such as the Rocky Mountains in Colorado, are known for their frequent afternoon thunderstorms. Keep in mind that if you can hear thunder, even if the sun is shining, you are in danger. Lightning can strike far from its originating cloud.

If your climate research indicates thunderstorms are typical where you will be hiking—such as the afternoon storms in Colorado—plan your itinerary to mitigate exposure to lightning. Prepare alternate routes that can take you down and around higher elevation areas in case of storms. Plan camps for lower elevations, and do not proceed into exposed terrain if you can hear thunder or see storm clouds approaching. If you are in an open area when a thunderstorm hits, get to safety as quickly as you can. Usually this means descending below the tree line. Exercise caution here if you descend off trail so that you don't get lost too. If descending below the tree line is not an option, you'll need to get as low as you can and minimize your contact with the ground. Use dips in the terrain and crouch down on tiptoe and on a foam sleeping pad if possible. The pad can help insulate you from indirect strikes. Be sure to remove as much metal from your person as possible, including zippers, the frame of your pack, trekking poles, jewelry, etc., and place it far away—at least 100 feet. However, if you're at risk of hypothermia or some other life-threatening situation, removing your rain jacket or other article of essential clothing because of a zipper is not a good idea. This is a scenario where you must do your best to triage the situation and mitigate as many risks as possible while staying as safe as you can. Be sure to position yourself 50 feet or more from other members of your party.

Heat and Heat Illness

At the beginning of this chapter, I mentioned my many close calls with dehydration and heat when I was first starting out hiking. Although it's not as dramatic as lightning, heat can be dangerous. There are various heat illnesses ranging from mild (heat rash) to life-threatening (heat stroke) that can happen to anyone during hot weather. Learning the symptoms and how to avoid and, if necessary, treat them can save your life on and off the trail.

Heat rash and heat cramps are quite common and result from exercising in heat and humidity. Losing fluids and salts while sweating is the cause of both of these conditions. They can

Katie Tip

When traveling in the backcountry, it's important to know your body, keep health conditions in mind, and have an understanding of how you react to different climates so that you can properly prepare. Not everyone reacts the same to hot, cold, wet, or dry conditions. For example, I run cold and have nerve damage in my hands from past frostbite. After more than enough instances of finding myself unprepared and in unnecessarily dangerous situations due to being overly cold, I now always carry hand warmers and a warmer sleeping bag than others might in the same conditions.

easily be prevented and treated by consuming adequate water and electrolytes as well as cooling off and/or resting in the shade.

The more serious heat illnesses are heat exhaustion and heat stroke. They also result from exercising in heat and humidity and losing too many fluids and salts through sweat, but they're more dangerous in that they can cause body temperature to rise to critical levels in a short period of time. In order to avoid these life-threatening illnesses, stay cool, stay hydrated, and maintain electrolyte balance. The safest thing you can do is to prevent heat stroke from happening.

While prevention is most desirable, knowing the symptoms of heat illnesses enables you to recognize and treat the conditions in their early stages. Make sure everyone in your party knows the symptoms and treatments for heat illnesses. Typically, symptoms progress from mild to severe, so the earlier you begin treatment, the better. Most heat illnesses start with heavy sweating followed by muscle cramping. The onset of headache, nausea, dizziness or fainting, shallow breathing, and/or a rapid and weak pulse can indicate heat exhaustion. When suffering from heat exhaustion, you're much more likely to have an accident, make a poor choice, or develop heat stroke. If you or another member of your party shows symptoms of heat exhaustion, it is imperative to cool down, hydrate, and rest.

When heat exhaustion is left unchecked, it can escalate into heat stroke, which is a medical emergency and needs to be treated by a medical professional. If you or a member of your party have the symptoms of heat exhaustion plus a temperature higher than 103 degrees Fahrenheit, flushed and/or hot and dry skin, a lack of sweating, slurred speech, or altered consciousness, you must utilize a PLB (see the section titled Personal Locator Beacons later in this chapter) or other communication device to call for help.

Dangers Associated with Cold Weather

The inverse of heat illness is what happens in cold weather. Long-term exposure to cold temperatures (especially if it's precipitating) can lead to frostbite and hypothermia, and both can be life-threatening. Frostbite is the freezing of your tissues; it generally occurs in extreme cold—below 32 degrees Fahrenheit—and is exacerbated by the wind. If you'll be hiking in these conditions, keeping all skin covered is very important. Any changes in skin color, temperature, or sensation are signs that you may be at risk of developing frostbite. If the frostbite is not stopped early and becomes severe enough, you may end up losing the affected part of the body and/or experience infections as the frozen tissue dies. As with heat illnesses, it's important to monitor your skin during cold-weather hiking and immediately take measures to mitigate the development of frostbite by getting warm and out of the elements.

Hypothermia is a condition that occurs when your body temperature drops too low. Unlike frostbite, extreme cold is not required, and precipitation is frequently a factor. Hypothermia is progressive, just like heat illnesses. If hypothermia is allowed to progress and your body temperature drops below 95 degrees, death is likely. Proper layering and avoiding getting wet in cold weather—either from sweat or precipitation—is essential to avoiding the development of hypothermia. If you notice the early signs of hypothermia—shivering, loss of energy, and/or growing sleepy—it's imperative to seek shelter, get dry, and warm up. Bear in mind that people experiencing hypothermia are often irrational and in a compromised mental state. Therefore, traveling in groups is one of the easiest ways to make traveling in cold weather safer. If you are alone, you may not recognize symptoms in yourself.

Katie Tip

In some situations, it may be necessary to use multiple methods of water treatment. On the Oregon Desert Trail, for example, where many of the water sources were cow tanks of varying levels of quality, there were times when I filtered water first through a bandana to remove sediment, then through a Sawyer Squeeze to remove bacteria and protozoa, and then treated it chemically because the source was so questionable. Carrying a couple of water-treatment methods can be useful to ensure you're removing all contaminants.

SNOW AND WATER

Water is a ubiquitous substance and while we need it to survive, it can also be a formidable force that can endanger backcountry hikers. In 2016, I set out to hike the 800-mile Arizona Trail. I started southbound in early October from the Utah border, headed to the Mexico border. The first day was perfect—sunny and warm. By midafternoon the second day, I was hiking through a snowstorm and in the early stages of hypothermia. When I woke up face-first in the snow and mud, I knew it was serious. I set up an emergency camp and did what I needed to do to regain body heat and survive.

For the majority of my Arizona Trail hike, I was primarily concerned about getting enough water. But on that afternoon in the slush and heavy snowfall, I wanted nothing to do with water, especially in its frozen form. In addition to protecting yourself in wet and snowy conditions, other important backcountry skills include fording potentially dangerous streams, using an ice axe, treating water for potability, and ensuring you drink enough.

Drinking Water

How much water you need to consume per day and, in conjunction, carry with you while backpacking is highly individualized and varies depending on conditions. There are risks associated with both having too much and having too little: Most people are familiar with dehydration, but it is also possible to drink too much, which can result in a condition called hyponatremia. This condition dilutes the salts in your body and in severe cases leads to death through tissue swelling.

Over time you'll learn how much water your body needs in various conditions; just remember, it's always safer to carry some extra water than to run out. However, if you'd like to get a more accurate base point prior to your long hike, you can calculate your sweat rate. It is a relatively easy process requiring a bathroom scale, some math, and the ability to exercise in similar conditions to those you'll encounter on your hike. There are many online calculators that can walk you through the process (see Additional Resources).

Another important aspect of hydration is ensuring that you have a way to treat your drinking water. Backcountry water can be contaminated with a wide range of bacteria, viruses, parasites, cysts, and other pathogens. In some areas it can also be contaminated with heavy metals, agricultural chemicals, or extractive industry compounds (from mining, etc.).

Not all water is contaminated to the same degree or by the same compounds. Most backcountry water in the United States can be adequately purified for drinking by using a water filter, chemical treatments (iodine, chlorine), boiling, or UV devices. Be aware, though, that not all of these methods remove all contaminants. It's good to know the limitations of your water-treatment system and pair the correct system with the types of water contaminants you anticipate along your route.

Fording

Sometimes your primary water concern in the backcountry has nothing to do with thirst. Unless you're hiking in an extremely arid or

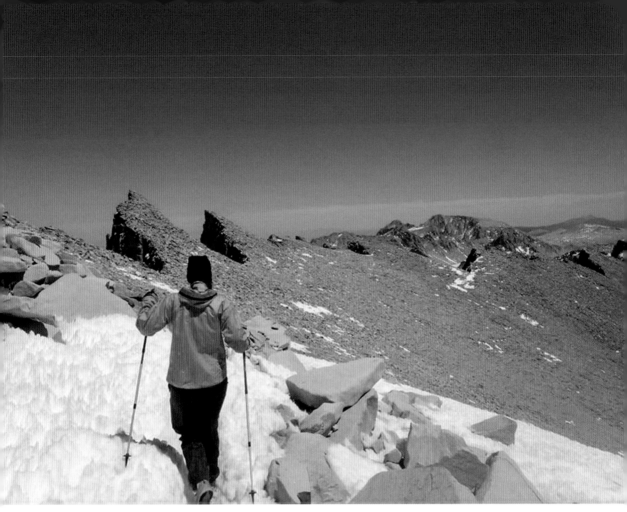

Descending Mount Whitney to return to the PCT

well-bridged landscape, you'll have to cross water. Usually, this isn't much of a problem aside from the annoyance of wet feet. Risks increase when water levels are high and/or there is a strong current, and when the water and/or ambient air temperatures are cold.

If you believe that fording poses a high risk, the safest thing you can do is turn around and go back. If this is not an option, be prepared to assess and mitigate the risk through a series of observations and fording techniques: First of all, check downstream for large rocks and rapids, waterfalls, fallen trees with branches in the water, or anything else that could trap you

or injure you if you fall in. It's also important to look at the embankments to see if you can get out easily. Second, look for wider areas where the current is less strong. Third, if you can see through the water examine the riverbed. You may be able to see deeper areas, hidden boulders, or other debris that you'll want to avoid. Most importantly, don't hesitate to search up- and downstream for a safer place to cross, and be sure to remain cognizant of where you are so you don't end up lost if you cross somewhere other than the trail crossing. No matter what methods or location you use for fording, always unclip the buckles of your pack so you can shed it easily if you fall in so it doesn't trap you.

In addition to the danger of drowning, hypothermia is a risk if you get soaked during your crossing. Falling in can also lead to the malfunction of electronics or destruction of paper navigational tools. Before plunging in, make sure that these important items are properly waterproofed and secured.

There are also many techniques for leveraging your other party members to cross water safely. While they are not discussed in this book, see Additional Resources to find further reading that goes in depth on this topic.

Snow and Ice

Many people are surprised to learn that in certain areas, snow may linger well into summer. Even in July you may encounter snow and ice across the trail in mountainous regions, especially in protected pockets. You may also encounter snow bridges across flowing water. At first glance they seem to be a solution to the fording risks previously discussed. However, if you choose to cross water on these bridges, be extremely careful as it can be difficult to evaluate the stability of a snow bridge; there is always a risk that it will collapse with you on it. This can lead to injury, entrapment, drowning, or hypothermia.

Any lingering snowpack from the previous winter can also pose other risks: the surface area of the snow is often hard and icy from having melted and refrozen many times throughout the winter, spring, and early summer, resulting in compromised traction even for boots with grippy soles. Sloped snow is even more precarious. To prepare to make these crossings safely, carry removable traction for your shoes, stability devices (trekking poles/whippet), and an ice axe. For trail hiking with occasional snow slopes, an ice axe is used for self-arrest and the occasional step chopping as opposed to

actual ice climbing. As with any tool, it's important to know how to properly use your traction devices, ice axe, and whippet. There are many online resources and in-person classes to help you learn proper techniques. See Additional Resources for suggestions. Since the purpose of

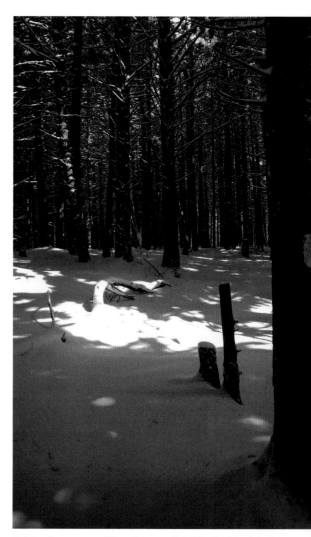

Cold and snowy conditions increase the risk of cold-related illnesses as well as navigational challenges.

THE TEN ESSENTIALS

The point of the Ten Essentials, originated by The Mountaineers, has always been to answer two basic questions: Can you prevent emergencies and respond positively should one occur (items 1–5)? And can you safely spend a night—or more—outside (items 6–10)? Use this list as a guide, and tailor it to the needs of your outing.

1. **Navigation:** The five fundamentals are a map, altimeter, compass, GPS device, and a personal locator beacon or other device to contact emergency first responders.
2. **Headlamp:** Include spare batteries.
3. **Sun protection:** Wear sunglasses, sun-protective clothes, and broad-spectrum sunscreen rated at least SPF 30.
4. **First aid:** Basics include bandages; skin closures; gauze pads and dressings; roller bandage or wrap; tape; antiseptic; blister prevention and treatment supplies; nitrile gloves; tweezers; needle; nonprescription painkillers; anti-inflammatory, anti-diarrheal, and antihistamine tablets; topical antibiotic; and any important personal prescriptions, including an EpiPen if you are allergic to bee or hornet venom.
5. **Knife:** Also consider a multitool, strong tape, some cordage, and gear repair supplies.
6. **Fire:** Carry at least one butane lighter (or waterproof matches) and firestarter, such as chemical heat tabs, cotton balls soaked in petroleum jelly, or commercially prepared firestarter.
7. **Shelter:** In addition to a rain shell, carry a single-use bivy sack, plastic tube tent, or jumbo plastic trash bag.
8. **Extra food:** For shorter trips a one-day supply is reasonable.
9. **Extra water:** Carry sufficient water and have the skills and tools required to obtain and purify additional water.
10. **Extra clothes:** Pack additional layers needed to survive the night in the worst conditions that your party may realistically encounter.

these devices is to dig in to hard, icy snow, they can all incur injury if used improperly. Practice with them as much as possible before use!

PHYSICAL PREPAREDNESS AND INJURY

Preparing your body for a long-distance hike is essential to a safe trip. Although accidents can occur despite your preparation and fitness, good decision-making, understanding your physical limits, and having the ability to treat injury in the field can make your trip a much safer experience.

For an in-depth discussion of how to prepare yourself physically for a long-distance hike, turn to chapter 7. Proper route selection based on physical condition is also addressed in that chapter. Appropriate conditioning and itinerary choices can greatly diminish injury risk in the backcountry. In this segment, we focus primarily on how to prevent and deal with injuries if they do occur.

Conditioning Injuries versus Accidents

Physical-injury risk factors can be divided into two broad categories: The first are injuries dependent on your physical conditioning, which is completely within your control. The second is accidental injury, which is not. Many people dismiss physical conditioning prior to a long-distance hike because they reason that they will "hike into shape." While this is basically true, it is also true that a structured training plan can ease your body's transition into full-time exercise, thus greatly decreasing your chance of an overuse injury.

Injury due to accidents is one of the least-avoidable risks we discuss in this chapter. Beyond proper conditioning and route selection, the guidance in this section can improve the overall outcomes of injuries when they occur. If you were to get into an accident or hurt yourself at home, you'd use the first-aid supplies you have on hand. If those were not enough to treat your injury, you'd seek professional medical attention. Your on- and off-trail safety protocols are not much different from one another. The biggest difference comes from ease and speed of implementation. Always carry a first-aid kit that can treat most minor injuries, equivalent to a medicine cabinet at home. This doesn't have to be elaborate (antibiotic ointment, bandages, pain relief medication, etc.). Having additional wilderness first-aid training (or the more extensive wilderness first responder course) can greatly assist you in your ability to decide what

to do in certain situations and which ones warrant emergency action. Even when you're on trail, if you're injured more severely than a medicine cabinet at home can treat, you need professional attention.

Personal Locator Beacons (PLBs)

In addition to having at least one person in your party with wilderness first-aid training or other formal professional medical expertise, carrying a PLB is also highly recommended.

PLBs such as SPOT or Garmin inReach are GPS-based devices that allow you to contact emergency services anywhere in the world by sending your precise coordinates to the nearest emergency personnel. Some of these devices also have built-in two-way communication systems so you can be in touch with loved ones no matter where you are. While they are excellent tools, especially in cases of emergency, they are not a replacement for good judgment. Ideally, a PLB is a piece of emergency gear that is always carried and never needed.

Wearing a medical ID bracelet or carrying a tag of some sort on your gear can assist rescue personnel in administering proper treatment to you in case you are found unconscious. This is especially important if you have allergies. You may consider also including your blood type and emergency contact numbers.

Remember, traveling with one or more partners can expedite receiving medical care in case of an injury. In a group of three or more, if one member of the party is immobilized, one person can remain with them while another goes for help. Be sure that all members know about allergies or prescriptions for other party members.

HUMAN INTERACTIONS

Of all the risks associated with backcountry travel, negative interactions with humans are the least predictable and potentially the most dangerous. However, these types of negative interactions are incredibly rare: the majority of people you meet in the outdoors are simply recreating. It is important to consider ways you will respond if potentially unsafe human interactions do occur, though. The following information is provided to get you started on your own thought experiments. Mentally rehearsing reactions to certain situations is a proven method for improving your overall response to those situations if and when they do occur. Turn to chapter 8 for more discussion on mental preparation.

Trust Your Gut

The simplest method for staying safe from humans is to trust your gut. It is also the method that is frequently ridiculed and socialized out of us. But like all animals, we have self-preservation instincts. Though there may be no overt words or actions to indicate that another human or situation is dangerous, if something feels off, pay attention to that nagging feeling. It is safer to remove yourself from a situation without reason than it is to wait and see if your gut was right. I'm sure I've left situations that would have turned out fine, but I'm happy I walked away. Being attuned to your body is important in more than just your physical training!

Lie if You Must

This recommendation shocks a lot of people. Remember, no one aside from your emergency contacts or land management agency needs to know where you're going or whether you are with other people. Questions about where you're camping and who you're with are common small-talk topics among long-distance hikers. However, if the person is pressing you for more details than you're comfortable sharing, consider that to be a red flag. In general, vague answers are usually safest and will satisfy the small-talk askers. If you begin to feel uncomfortable with a conversation, it is OK to tell them directly that you don't want to answer their question or,

if necessary, lie and remove yourself from the situation as quickly as possible. Again, trust your instincts.

Camp Discreetly

We are the most vulnerable while we sleep. In addition to choosing a campsite that is safe from weather, selecting a discreet site can mitigate potentially dangerous interactions with other humans. Camp well off trail, preferably out of sight, following Leave No Trace ethics (see "The Seven Principles of Leave No Trace" sidebar in chapter 2). Don't camp near a road or a place where people obviously party, ride ATVs, or engage in any other non-human-powered activity.

Carry Protection

Weapons are very controversial in the hiking world, but guns and knives are not the only forms of protection that you can potentially carry: Many nonlethal methods, such as bear mace or wasp spray, work on animals of both the two- and four-legged variety. And the most important weapon you carry is always your brain.

Katie Tip

Like Heather, I never question my gut instinct, especially on trail. If a situation or person raises even the slightest red flag for me, I don't hesitate to lie, answer vaguely, and extract myself from the situation as quickly as possible. The subconscious mind often picks up on clues that your conscious mind can't pinpoint. You don't need a logical reason, and you don't need to be "polite" the way society trains us to be. Your priority is your safety. Your intuition and instincts are always speaking to you. Hearing that inner voice and trusting it is a muscle that can be strengthened. If listening to and trusting those nudges is foreign to you, begin practicing now, before you even set foot in the wilderness.

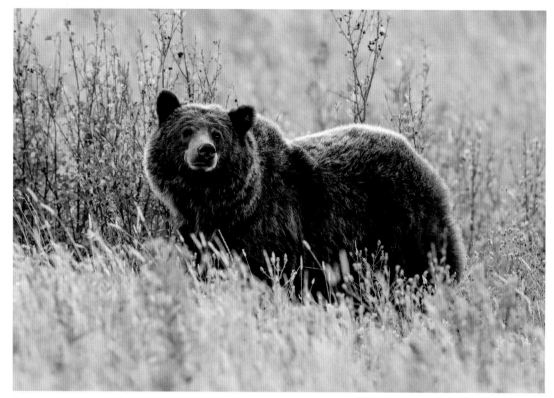

Seeing a grizzly bear in the wild can be exhilarating—and potentially hazardous. (Photo by Frank Fichtmueller)

ANIMAL INTERACTIONS

We have finally arrived at bears, the topic that opened this chapter. Many years ago, I worked as a seasonal employee for the National Park Service at Glacier National Park in Montana. As you may know, Glacier—and the ribbon of protected lands connecting it to Yellowstone National Park—supports the largest population of grizzly bears in the Lower 48. During my summer of hiking there, I covered more than 400 backcountry miles. All but about 50 miles of them were solo.

"Aren't you afraid of bears?" people would ask.

No. I respected that there were a lot of bears there, both grizzly and black. I accepted the increased risks associated with hiking solo (discussed more in the next section), and I learned everything I could about bears and bear behavior. I equipped myself with knowledge of how to respond in an encounter with a large member of the *Ursus* genus.

So when I came around a corner on trail in late August and found myself eye-to-eye with a sow grizzly and her two cubs, I reacted instantly. I broke eye contact, yielded ground, prepared my bear spray, and waited for her to make her decision. To date, the following ten minutes were some of the more frightening and also spellbinding of my entire life. I am thankful that in that situation, she opted not to attack in defense of her cubs and eventually moved off the trail, allowing me to pass.

While I fully realize that this encounter could have gone another way, I do believe that animals inherently want to avoid humans. Recognizing that fact can help you overcome any irrational fear of animals, a fear that can be incapacitating to some—even to the point of keeping them home. Educating yourself about the animals you're likely to encounter on your route can help you prepare for possible interactions so that—like human encounters—you can react swiftly, which may keep you safer.

Campsite Evaluation

Proper campsite selection can also keep you safer from animal encounters. Camping near water sources, for example, increases the probability that animals will enter or come close to your site. Even if those animals are harmless, their predators may follow! Before setting up camp, take note of any large quantities of scat and/or game trails in the area. These are clear indicators that animals use this space and that you'll be placing yourself directly in their path.

Habituated versus Wild Animals

One factor that is out of your control is the habituation of animals you encounter. Any time a wild animal becomes comfortable near humans, it is considered to be habituated. Wildlife that is not habituated generally wants to get away from you as quickly as possible. Often you won't even see these animals. Think about birds: you can't easily catch a wild bird. However, birds that live near popular trails or city parks that are frequently hand-fed may not only come to you if asked but harass you until you give them a snack! This behavior extends to animals such as chipmunks, birds, and—you guessed it—bears that have received food directly or indirectly from people. Many hikers have been harassed by a chipmunk or a gray jay while taking a break. It's cute at first but quickly becomes annoying, and you may even find yourself tossing a bite of your snack their way so that they'll leave you and your gear alone. Now, imagine the animal seeking food is a bear. That is a much bigger problem.

And it isn't just food that determines habituation: Urban sprawl and increased human use of certain areas often bring humans and animals closer together than animals would like. Their options are to move out of their terrain or learn to deal with having humans close by. This proximity adjustment can lead to conflict.

When planning your hike, keep in mind the types of animals you may run into. If possible, avoid camping or taking extended breaks in areas with habituated wildlife. Many land management agencies publish these areas, but you can also assess the animals and the circumstances in which you meet them on your own.

Providing Ample Space

Every animal has a personal space bubble. In general, the bigger the animal, the bigger this bubble. Do your best to stay outside an animal's personal space bubble at all times. You may need to back up or go around them, especially if they don't have easy access to an escape route. Most of the time, animals will see, hear, or smell you coming and flee before you even see them, but sometimes the terrain may block their retreat so their only way out is right where you are standing. I once came across a herd of bighorn sheep high up near Swiftcurrent Pass on the CDT. Unfortunately, the ram determined I was a threat and began advancing toward me—head lowered. To my right was a sheer rock face, to the left a several-thousand-foot drop-off. I had no choice but to hurriedly back up on the trail until he stopped. Thankfully the entire herd fled up the cliff face, and I was able to continue safely on my way. But it was a terrifying few moments! When you encounter an animal, rapidly assess whether it has the ability to get away from you or not. Do what you can to optimize the space between you.

Wild animals live in a world without medical interventions. Injuries, even minor ones, often mean death from subsequent infection. Since most wild animals view humans as apex predators, they are unlikely to see you as a source of food (although habituated ones might), and they will do anything to get away from you and avoid injury. However, a mama bear is a classic example of an animal that attacks in defense rather than for food. In general, mothers with young are much more likely to attack if they feel their offspring are threatened. Even herbivores may take action to protect their young. Retreat is the best option whenever you are in this situation.

For additional in-depth information about how to respond in encounters with various animals, see Additional Resources or the complementary Backpacker Academy online course.

Domesticated Animals

The most frequently encountered dangerous animal I've experienced on trail is the domestic dog. Domestic dogs have complex psychology, which varies widely, making them much harder to predict. If you choose to hike with a canine companion, it is essential—and usually the law—for it to be on a leash at all times. This is for the safety of other hikers, the native wildlife, and your dog.

But what about other people's dogs that might be off-leash on trail? I've had success with these tactics:

- If the dog is barking but not approaching, stop and call out for an owner and request they leash their dog. If an owner does not appear, or if they refuse to catch hold of their dog, treat it as you would a wild animal.
- Give the dog space and try to de-escalate until the situation resolves (owner appears, dog leaves, or you are able to choose an alternate path around).
- If a dog attacks, fight back. Even smaller dogs have the ability and instinct to kill. Always protect your neck and stay on your feet.

- Report any dog attacks to authorities. Attempt to gather and relay owner information if you can safely do so. Be sure to ascertain whether the animal has had its rabies vaccine and seek medical attention for any bites.

RISK FACTORS ASSOCIATED WITH SOLO BACKCOUNTRY TRAVEL

It is often said that solo backpacking is the most dangerous. This is undeniably true, and from a safety standpoint, solo backcountry travel is not recommended. However, solitude in nature can also be extremely rewarding, and many people will choose that experience. Personally, I have covered tens of thousands of backcountry miles solo in terrain all over the United States, from the Sonoran Desert to the North Cascades, the Rocky Mountains to the boglands of Maine. I have had close calls with every single topic we've covered in this chapter. But I've also become a strong, independent, and risk-averse hiker and climber through critical thinking, experiences, and learning. The goal of this entire chapter is to set you on your own path of learning, thinking, and preparing to reduce risk and have an enjoyable experience in the backcountry, alone or with others.

If you choose to backpack solo, do not downplay the risks associated with it. Accept them, take them seriously, and prepare for them. All the risks covered in this chapter become even more dangerous if you are facing them alone. Crossing strong water without a partner results in a higher likelihood of being swept off your feet. Encountering dangerous wildlife alone makes you more vulnerable than when you're part of a group. Individuals are a target for human violence at a much higher rate than groups are. If you are injured or are succumbing to heat or cold illness alone, you have to recognize what has happened and treat yourself. These are serious risks that need to be addressed in your planning and preparation.

Each individual's tolerance for risk is different. Over time, you'll learn your personal risk tolerance. As a result of some dangerous experiences, I've become less risk tolerant in many situations. In others, I have gained enough skills that I've become more risk tolerant. The most crucial thing I have learned to do when hiking solo is to stop and turn back. Many deaths occur in the backcountry due to people pushing past their limits into situations they are not equipped for. Do not become one of these statistics. Instead, if you choose to go solo, spend time in your planning process considering what risks are likely and how to handle them and at what point you will turn back or take an alternate route. The Assessing Risk Checklist at the end of this book can guide you in this effort.

It's essential to leave an itinerary and emergency contact with a responsible person whom you trust. Again, there is a sample worksheet at the end of this book to help you.

Before venturing out solo, take the time to build your backpacking skills slowly and safely. Make sure you have mastered navigation, first aid, assessment of water and snow risks, each item of gear, campsite selection, proper animal encounter etiquette, and the knowledge of how your body responds to heat, cold, altitude, and climatic shifts.

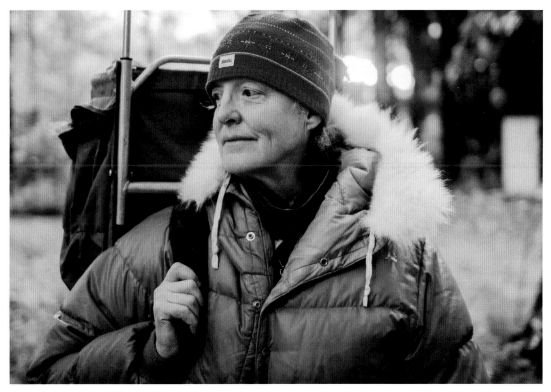

Carolyn "Ravensong" Burkhart, the first woman to solo thru-hike the PCT, modeling the gear she used in 1976 (Photo by Tommy Corey)

4

NAVIGATION & ROUTE PREPAREDNESS

BY *Heather*

In 2006, I set out with my partner at the time to thru-hike the CDT from Canada to Mexico through the wild landscapes of Montana, Idaho, Wyoming, Colorado, and New Mexico. GPS units back then were rudimentary and expensive, so instead, we carried multiple sets of maps and our compass. Although we had basic map and compass skills, it was still a steep learning curve finding our way along a mostly unmarked and unbuilt route. One day as we made our way along the wide-open ridgelines of Montana, we stopped to review our maps. My partner pointed to a ridge leading away from the one we were on and identified it as the correct one to follow.

Thirty minutes and several hundred feet of elevation loss later, we stopped. The slope of the ridgeline we'd descended had been steep, loose, and full of krummholz that tore at our skin, clothes, and gear. We reconvened around the map, this time orienting it with our compass only to discover that we'd been on the correct ridge earlier after all! Thus, we began the difficult slog back up the slope we'd just gone down. We learned a valuable lesson that day: without a compass, maps are not effective navigational tools. Orienting your map, or otherwise pinpointing your location with accuracy before making a route decision, is critical to staying on route and safe in the backcountry.

Unlike the weather, staying found in the backcountry is completely within your control! Mitigate the risks of getting lost with proper knowledge of how to use navigational tools, good decision-making, and a well-constructed (and frequently referenced) beta packet.

NAVIGATIONAL TOOLS

This section covers the practical navigational techniques most commonly needed and used on long-distance trails, such as trail-specific apps. While we briefly address basic map and compass skills, it's beyond the scope of this book to provide thorough training with regard to their use. Mastering map and compass skills requires practice, and these skills are best learned through hands-on or video education. There are many resources online or at outdoor retailers that can give you focused training in these techniques. We also offer in-depth map, compass, and GPS training in the Backpacker Academy navigation course.

These days I use GPS technology as my primary navigational tool. Like many hikers, I find that the ease of use and accuracy make it the best option. However, I also reference print maps and carry a compass. Knowing the strengths, weaknesses, and proper applications of various navigational tools is an important part of traveling in the backcountry.

No matter what tools you are using, keep in mind that rushed choices are often the ones that lead to errors. Back when my partner and I were standing on that Montana ridgeline, the weather was tanking. It was cold, windy,

and we wanted to be anywhere but high and exposed. Instead of layering up and taking the time to orient our map correctly, we gave it a cursory glance, decided that the lower, tree-covered ridge was the right one . . . and went for it. It's important to always orient your map, consult your beta packet, and use your GPS or otherwise verify your location before making a decision. Errors like this might simply result in a few "bonus miles," but they can also result in more serious situations. Resist the urge to make rash navigational decisions because of extenuating factors (impending weather or darkness, the need to reach town by a certain time, etc.).

Map and Compass

As mentioned, paper maps should always be used in conjunction with a compass. It's tempting to make the terrain match the map, rather than match the map to the terrain, especially when you're fatigued or stressed, but using a compass to accurately orient your map greatly reduces the risk of mismatching the two. There are a few techniques you'll need to understand in order to use a map and compass for on-trail navigation:

- How compasses work
- How to use a topographical map
- How to orient a map

In addition, always protect your maps by either using waterproof maps or carrying them in a waterproof case. Also, ensure that you keep your maps and compass in a secure location where they can't fall out or get snagged on a bush and be lost.

How Compasses Work

Compasses detect the magnetic field of the earth. The needle of the compass is attracted to the *magnetic* North Pole (more on this later), not the physical North Pole, through magnetization. In many ways, compasses function very simply, yet the magnetic field of the earth itself is still not completely understood. In fact, there is some level of disagreement on why the magnetic field exists at all! Even the polarity will shift at some point as it has many times in the past—meaning that compass needles would then point to the South Pole rather than the North.

Keep in mind that the magnetic field of the earth is not centered at the North Pole. The magnetic field emanates from the middle of the planet and is vertical at the poles, with the North Pole currently operating as a southern polarity

> **Katie Tip**
>
> *Like Heather, I rely on GPS as my primary navigation tool. However, I also carry paper maps and a compass every time I go on a multi-night backpacking trip. Those tools are only worth the extra pack weight if you know how to use them, of course, and I've found that the best way to improve map and compass skills is to practice in the field, in low risk situations. For that reason, I frequently reference what I see in the field with what's on my map and I practice skills like taking a bearing in the field and transferring it to a map. Using paper maps provides more context than a small GPS screen and allows me to better understand the topography through which I'm traveling. I also appreciate the peace of mind of having analog backups if my GPS breaks, fails, or is lost, which is not uncommon with electronics.*

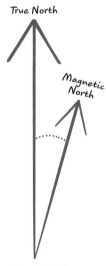

Declination		[X]
Model Used:	WMM-2020	
Latitude:	39.0968° N	ⓘ
Longitude:	120.0324° W	
Date	**Declination**	
2021-0_-_5	13.11° E ± 0.36° changing by 0.09° W per year	

True North

Magnetic North

Mount Rainier National Park

Declination varies by location.

and therefore attracting the northern polarity of your compass needle.

Think back to science class. Did you ever have dipole magnets that you simply could not force together? Then you swapped one around and they instantly slammed together and were hard to pry apart? The ends of those magnets were marked with *N* and *S*—the same as the poles of our planet.

To understand how navigational methods such as compasses, datums, and GPS technology work, it helps to understand a bit about our planet. The earth is a three-dimensional—yet not perfect—sphere called an oblate spheroid or oblate ellipsoid. Therefore, all systems of navigation and measurement must use triangulation or other methods to delineate your location on the spheroid. In addition, your use of a compass is affected by the fact that magnetic north is constantly moving while physical north (true north) remains constant; this angle of difference is referred to as declination.

Declination changes at a variable rate as the magnetic-field-generating core of the earth shifts. It is critical to set your declination properly before every major trip and understand that even if you never leave your region, you will need to reset it on a regular basis. Declination is monitored in the United States by NOAA, the same agency we've referred you to for weather research. You can consult them (or countless other online sources) to determine what the declination is for where you will be backpacking. Most compasses come with instructions on how to set declination and it usually requires a built-in tool. Because declination is *always* changing, you will need to look up the current declination even if your map has declination printed on it. Declination is also the reason that navigating by compass at high and low latitudes becomes very imprecise.

Anatomy of a Compass

The basic parts of a compass that you'll need to know are the baseplate, direction-of-travel arrow, markings for measuring, needle, bezel, orientation lines, orientation arrow, and declination adjuster.

How to Choose a Map

For all backcountry trips make sure you choose a detailed topographic map. Visitor-center–style maps are *not* appropriate for navigation, even if they show trails. These types of maps are often not drawn to scale and don't include topographic lines. Therefore, if you get off trail or aren't sure where you are, it will be impossible to orient yourself. Topographic maps indicate landforms with the use of contour lines (relief), water features (hydrography), and tree cover through shading. Each of these along with manmade (buildings, roads, boundaries, etc.) and toponymic (place name) features is useful for navigation. Choose a topographical map that is drawn "to scale" meaning that it accurately translates the three-dimensional earth into a two-dimensional format. When paired with a compass set with proper declination, these maps are good tools for backcountry navigation.

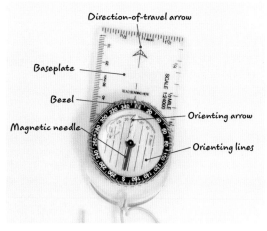

The basic features of a compass (declination adjuster on back)

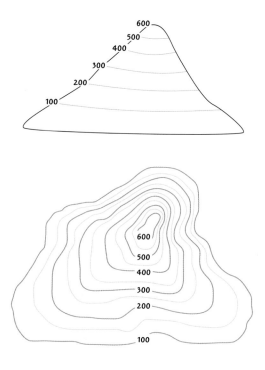

A simple illustration of the principles of contour lines to represent three-dimensional terrain

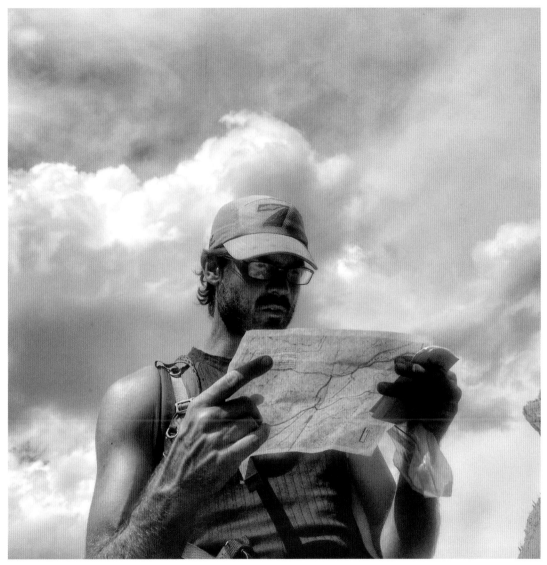

Knowing how to read a topographic map is crucial.

Anatomy of a Topographical Map

Lines on a topographical map are made by connecting points on the map that are the same elevation. Therefore, lines that are closer together indicate steep terrain. Topographic lines that are spaced farther apart indicate a mellower slope. These lines are labeled by their elevation, although most maps will not label every one but will only label lines every hundred, couple hundred, or thousand feet. The interval of each topographic line can be determined by dividing the difference between two labeled lines by the number of intervening lines. Keep in mind that features at or between the interval will not be represented as a distinct feature on the map. Comparing the labeled lines near one another is how you determine if the elevation is going up or down on a particular feature.

How to Orient the Map

Once you have the topographical map for your hike and your compass declination set for the area, you are ready to use the map and compass together to navigate. The first step in this pairing is orienting the map. Once the map is oriented, you can compare it to your surroundings and make your navigational decisions.

The first step is to place your compass flat on the map. You can do this on your palm or a rock or even the ground. It's important to keep them level and align the straight edge of the compass with one of the straight edges of the map, making sure the compasses direction-of-travel arrow (which is painted on the baseplate) is pointing toward the top of the map.

Next, you'll rotate the bezel until the N is lined up with the direction-of-travel arrow.

Finally, you'll need to rotate everything together, including your body. If you use the ground or a rock, carefully pick everything up without losing alignment. Turn until the needle is aligned with the orientation needle. Now your map is oriented, as are you, and you can navigate accurately.

Satellite Technology

There are many different satellite-positioning systems in orbit around the earth. GPS is a satellite-positioning constellation owned and operated by the United States government. GPS has become a generic term for the use of satellite technology even if the data is coming from another network. Throughout this book, GPS is

Katie Tip

In addition to your map and compass, GPS apps can be a useful navigational tool for long-distance hikes as well as for planning and tracking routes locally and in new locations. Apps such as Gaia GPS and CalTopo offer a variety of map layers (e.g., USFS maps, air quality, cell coverage, NatGeo Trails Illustrated, Native Land Territories, weather overlays, etc.) that can be used together to create an informative and comprehensive understanding of the area you're traveling through. As Heather mentions, the most important thing to remember is to download the maps of your route and the surrounding corridor ahead of time, while you still have internet access. Here's a reliable way to test whether your maps are downloaded for offline use: Clear the app cache, switch your phone to airplane mode, and open the app. Can you see your maps in detail?

used in this generic sense. Unlike a compass, you do not have to adjust GPS for declination or orient it to your map, generally making it a more efficient method of navigation. Mapping apps that you use on your phone to drive from point A to point B use satellite technology. Your GPS receiver of choice can place you on the surface of the earth, and at your altitude above the surface with great precision. There are two types of GPS receivers that most people consider for their backcountry navigational purposes: standalone devices and smartphone apps.

Standalone GPS Devices

You may be familiar with what are commonly referred to as GPS units. In many outdoor stores there are displays of multiple makes and models. Some have additional features beyond navigation, including cameras and removable storage. They also vary as to their screen size, color options, and other specs. Provided that your device comes with maps, or you have actively uploaded the maps, use is fairly straightforward. When you look at the screen, you will see an indicator of your current location. From there you will be able to toggle and zoom to see map information relative to your location. For many years these standalone devices were the only option if you wanted to use satellite navigation in the backcountry.

Chapter 3, on backcountry safety, mentions the importance of carrying a PLB, and although PLBs do not offer any navigational capabilities, they do use satellite-positioning networks similar to your navigational GPS devices. This is why, when you activate a PLB, emergency personnel receive accurate coordinates of your location. This method of information transfer is a huge advancement in the world of search and rescue.

GPS Apps

The navigational method used most commonly among long-distance backpackers is a GPS-based app on their smartphone. This application is superior both to a map and compass due to the accuracy of satellite navigation and to standalone GPS units because most hikers are already carrying their phones.

There are a variety of options, and I discuss the two most popular in a bit more detail here. Most apps are extremely user friendly with short learning curves, although you'll want to familiarize yourself with them prior to setting out. Keep in mind that you may need to load the base maps in the app you're using. You'll also need to carry a backup map and compass as well as have a plan for both protecting/waterproofing and charging your phone.

General Navigation Apps

There are many navigational apps available on the market. The one that I have used for regions not covered by trail-specific apps (see next section) is Gaia GPS. Gaia (and other apps like it) allows for several different base-map options and you can easily plot a route, import routes and waypoints from other sources, and create a tracklog of your

trip. Though it is a phone app, it functions offline. However, the downloading of maps must be done while you are connected to the internet.

Trail-Specific Apps

The most popular app among long-distance hikers for trail-specific navigation is the Farout (from Atlas Guides) series. They produce detailed navigational information for numerous trails and trail systems on multiple continents. In addition to providing a base map and a location, they also show track lines for the trail you are hiking as well as popular side trails, elevation profiles, and waypoints (camping areas, water sources, etc.). These waypoints also have commenting areas, where fellow app-using hikers can communicate things such as water quality, hazards, and other pertinent information.

These apps offer navigation and more, enabling you to not only find where you are and where you're going but research what to expect when you get there. Another benefit for hikes on long-distance trails, such as the PCT, is that town information is supplied, which can help you find what you need easily when you reach your resupply point. You can also use their route building tools to plan your trip in detail based on elevation, water, and camping. In addition, an integrated check-in feature can be used to stay in touch with family and friends while you're hiking. Please note that at the time of this writing, the feature relies on connectivity to transmit check-ins (though you can initiate them anytime), so it is not for use in emergencies.

As with Gaia, the app functions fully offline, though initial app setup and the loading of maps must be done while connected to the internet.

THE BETA PACKET

The more familiar you are with your route; the easier navigation will be. Familiarize yourself with things such as general terrain, water features, type of trail bed, alternate and emergency routes along the way, and locations/descriptions of potentially confusing junctions. But how can you know all of this for a long-distance route? Or for a trail you've never traveled? Compile a beta packet—a selection of reference materials—for your route.

Guidebooks, trip reports from blogs or other online resources, detailed topographic maps, and images from route descriptions are all excellent ways to familiarize yourself with the hike you'll be taking. Depending on your trek, you may want to carry some combination of these

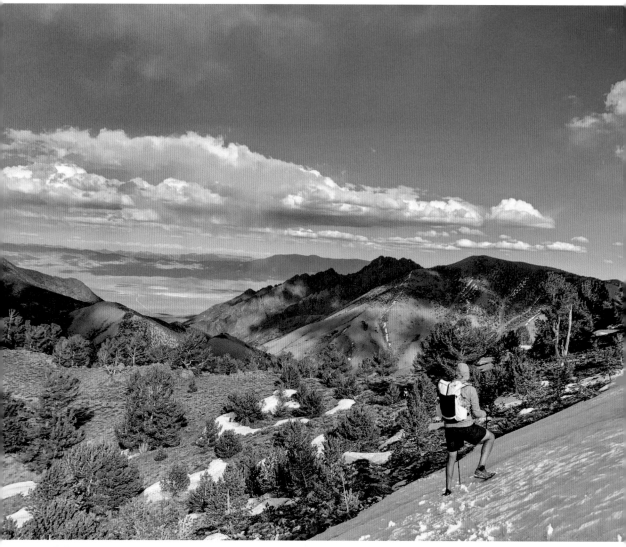

Taking in ridge line views and pondering the vastness of the Great Basin

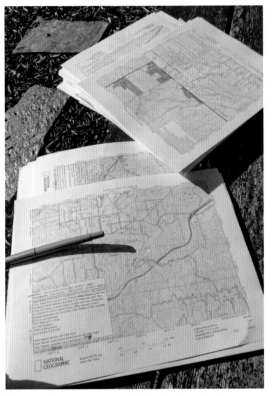

Topographic maps are essential for backcountry travel.

my second PCT hike, I realized I'd made a wrong turn when I came to a lovely creek in the middle of what was supposed to be a waterless stretch. While on your hike, review the day ahead each evening or first thing in the morning to refresh your mind.

Alternate routes are an important part of any beta packet because there are times when things go wrong due to weather, injury, or other unexpected challenges. For shorter trips, it's possible to note these options on your maps from home, but for longer journeys, such as the PCT or AT, it's impossible to research everything from home. While trail-specific apps such as Farout are incredibly detailed for the trail corridor itself, the base maps often do not show farther than a few miles out. Therefore, if you need to exit the trail for some reason, you will need another reference. Wider topographic or DeLorme Atlas–type maps can be helpful, or you can also have the maps of the region in a non-trail-specific app or GPS (such as Gaia GPS). For areas where bad weather and precarious terrain are common (such as in the High Sierra or Glacier Peak Wilderness on the PCT or the White Mountains on the AT), it is a good idea to research some options from home and have alternates in mind in case of need. Many long-distance hikers are amazed to find out how close they are to a road even in the midst of these seemingly vast wilderness areas.

Backpacking requires constant peripheral attention to and often focused attention on your location in relation to where you've been and where you are going. There are many tools available that can help keep you on route. These range from higher-tech options, such as GPS and navigation apps, to paper maps, compasses, and other print materials. No matter which combination you choose, learn to rely on your tools and reference them often. The most important part of backcountry travel is arriving safely back in civilization at the end of your trip.

with you (either in paper or digital format); this makes up your beta packet, which you'll want to be familiar with before you depart and also review regularly en route. This will help you stay found, rather than trying to get un-lost.

For each day of your trip, use your map and resources from your beta packet to plan your day. Make notes of things like water sources (and the distance between them), hazards (deep water fords, exposed terrain, etc.), and type of trail tread (which can impact your hiking pace). These factors will play into your pace, pack weight, and potential camping areas, and they can play a role in helping you navigate. Knowing what to expect that day can help you notice a navigational error sooner rather than later. On

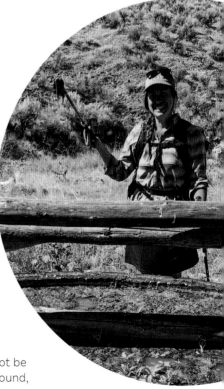

5

CREATING A RESILIENT BODY

BY *Katie*

Have you ever seen those photo series that depict how hikers' bodies change over the course of a thru-hike? A distinct transformation unfolds, and it becomes more dramatic the longer a hiker is on trail: By the end of a trip, their eyes have a distant gaze and the facial expression is one of genuine contentment. Their bodies are leaner and stronger. And although fitness levels undoubtedly improve, hikers all too often finish their trips gaunt and depleted.

A long-distance hike demands more of the human body than most athletic endeavors. Not only are you commonly hiking ten or more hours daily but you're doing that day after day for months. You are faced with strenuous climbs, rough terrain, exposure to heat and cold, ridgetop rains, and desert dryness. Your body has just a small amount of time to recover while you sleep before you demand more of it again. You may not be sleeping well on that thin layer of foam between you and the ground, and due to constraints inherent to backpacking, your diet is not optimal for glowing health (though this book will help with that!). In short, a long hike taxes the body, and you'll face an uphill battle if you embark on your journey in an already depleted state. I've witnessed many hikers suffer from extreme fatigue, illness, and injury that decreased the enjoyment of their hike or sent them home early. But this wear and tear on the body can be mitigated by bolstering your health in the months leading up to your adventure. The key is to create a resilient body, one that has reserves to draw on and can withstand hardship and recover quickly. Because on a long hike, you *will* face obstacles, both mentally and physically. This chapter and the following two cover physical preparation; mental preparation is covered in chapter 8. To dive more deeply into the application of these principles on building resilient health before your hike, consider our complementary Adventure Ready online course (see Additional Resources).

HOW RESILIENT HEALTH IMPACTS YOUR BACKPACKING TRIP

Resilience is the ability to withstand or quickly recover from adversity and difficult situations. A healthy, nourished, and well-trained body is a resilient body. A depleted body, on the other hand, becomes ill more easily and is slower to recover. Depletion occurs when there are more demands than the body can keep up with. The body's ability to keep up with physical and mental demands depends on getting adequate rest and nourishment and reducing sources of inflammation. In this chapter, we look at common sources of inflammation, how inflammation undermines optimal health, and how you can design a lifestyle that reduces it. To read more about nourishment, turn to chapter 6.

As you read this chapter, remember that everyone is unique, and what works for one person may not work for another. Though our

Heather Tip

Are women better suited to long-distance backpacking? This is a question I've been asked, and I've seen it stated as fact, often because of before-and-after pictures in which men often look emaciated and women frequently look strong. However, I don't believe that one gender or another is better suited to the rigors of the trail. Instead, there are differences in the ways male and female bodies react to the stress of backpacking as well as individual differences. Preparing for and knowing how your body responds to these stressors can help you stay strong from start to finish.

recommendations are based on peer-reviewed science, you must be the expert on your own body. If you choose to implement any of the lifestyle shifts described here, observe the results and make decisions accordingly.

Inflammation and Peak Performance

Most likely you've heard about inflammation, but what is it actually? And why, as a hiker, do you care? Inflammation is a natural and essential part of the immune system that allows the body to heal damaged areas and defend against foreign invaders. Acute inflammation, for example, is the redness and swelling that occurs at the site of an injury, causing a rush of pro-inflammatory cells that prevent infection and allow healing to take place. Without it, we wouldn't last long.

Problems arise when the source of the inflammation is persistent and the inflammatory response gets stuck in the "on" position. This is called chronic inflammation, and it's what we're referring to when we speak of the deleterious effects of inflammation throughout this book. It causes the immune system to become overactive, spreading inflammation throughout the body. Chronic inflammation manifests differently for everyone, but it tends to develop in the following areas: the brain and nervous system, digestive tract, detoxification system, endocrine system, musculoskeletal system, and immune system. Symptoms range from mild to severe. Milder symptoms include joint pain, fatigue, mood disorders, gastrointestinal complications, and weight fluctuations. On the more severe side of the inflammation continuum is our modern chronic illness epidemic, which affects more than 60 percent of American adults with ailments like cardiovascular disease, type 2 diabetes, autoimmune diseases, and Alzheimer's.

When inflammation is high and persistent, it affects all body systems and thus can affect your peak performance on trail. It contributes to decreased energy and endurance and undermines your body's ability to recover and repair quickly. It reduces immune system strength, which slows wound healing, causing you to feel run-down, and putting you at risk for more frequent illness. Inflammation can cause joint aches, stiffness that doesn't subside, and a general feeling of lethargy. Talk about a buzzkill when you're out trying to enjoy nature! The good news is that once you're aware of the sources, there are actions you can take to protect your health.

The remainder of this chapter outlines methods for reducing systemic inflammation so that you can hit the trail feeling as strong as possible. Chronic inflammation can be reduced and health resiliency built through dietary changes (covered in chapter 6), optimizing your gut health, prioritizing sleep, stressing less, spending time outside, and supplementing wisely.

Sources of Inflammation

In the modern world, sources of inflammation are unfortunately ubiquitous, and intentional effort is required to mitigate or avoid them. Fortunately, most sources of inflammation are under your control. Some common sources include dietary triggers (see chapter 6), gut dysbiosis (microbial imbalance), poor sleep, stress, social isolation, and environmental toxins. In athletes, the harmful effects of persistent inflammation can also occur from overtraining, which leads to compromised performance and immunity.

Debunking Vitamin I

If you hang out in the long-distance hiking community, you'll hear hikers talk about "vitamin I." This refers to the unfortunate habit many hikers have of relying on ibuprofen to get them through each day. When I was hiking the AT before ultralight gear was as prevalent as it is now and hikers' packs were heavier (on average), it was not uncommon to hear about hikers taking ibuprofen with breakfast, lunch, and dinner just to make it through the day—every day. While non-steroidal anti-inflammatory drugs (NSAIDs), such as ibuprofen, may provide temporary relief, chronic use has been associated with bleeding in the stomach and bowels as well as kidney and liver damage. NSAIDs can help in an acute situation, such as if you sprain an ankle and need to hike out to safety, but ultimately, they mask the message your body is communicating with you. Consistent pain and discomfort is your body's way of saying that it's overworked and it needs time to rest and repair. Ignoring this message can result in hike-ending overuse injuries and tissue damage that can take months (or years) to repair after your hike. Using natural methods to reduce inflammation, as outlined in this chapter, is a safer and more sustainable approach.

OPTIMIZING YOUR GUT HEALTH

"All disease begins in the gut." This oft-cited quote is attributed to the ancient Greek physician Hippocrates. More than two thousand years after the father of medicine made this observation, the study of the microbiome—the aggregate of microbiota that live in and on the human body and outnumber human cells ten to one—is one of the most rapidly growing fields of research. New studies illuminate the impact of the microbiome on almost every aspect of human health, from immune function to mood, brain health, and beyond. In this section, learn to recognize signs that your gut may need some attention and use best practices to get it functioning optimally.

Your gut health influences your entire body, contributing to a strong immune system, a healthy heart, optimal brain function, improved mood, good sleep, effective digestion, and even the prevention of chronic disease—all of which is essential for an enjoyable backpacking trip! A well-functioning digestive system is responsible for optimal nutrient absorption, proper energy production, metabolism, and elimination of toxins and other waste products. Repairing the gut can resolve food intolerances and clear up troublesome symptoms such as joint pain, digestive issues, brain fog, hormone imbalances, and much more. But it's not always obvious when your gut health is suffering as many signs are subtle. Keep an eye out for the following: food intolerances, weight-loss resistance, erratic or unstable moods, brain fog, fatigue, auto-immunity, skin irritation, sleep disturbances, and hormonal imbalances. Other issues to be aware of are digestive disturbances like gas, bloating, constipation, diarrhea, and heartburn. Fortunately, there are ways to heal the gut using dietary changes and supplementation, for example, which can result in a big shift in how you feel and your overall level of health.

Creating and Maintaining Gut Health

The key to gut health is having a large number and diversity of beneficial microbes. Creating and maintaining a healthy gut is similar to growing a healthy garden: just as a gardener creates an appropriate environment, plants seeds, and then nurtures the growing seedlings with water and nutrients, you can optimize your gut health by creating a suitable environment for microbes to thrive, inoculating the gut with a wide variety of microbes, and feeding the microbiota what they need to thrive. This approach is known as the seed-and-feed strategy. The microbes you use to seed your gut are probiotics: live bacteria and yeasts that are found naturally in certain foods. When consumed, probiotics colonize your gut and provide health benefits to you, the host. The nutrients you use to feed the microbiota are prebiotics: a type of fiber that is nondigestible.

Contrary to popular belief, probiotic supplements alone do not ensure good gut health. You could consume a whole bottle of probiotics, but if you're not eating the right foods to feed those probiotics, then you won't be able to maintain a healthy population. Furthermore, some foods and lifestyle practices can harm your microbiome, and no amount of probiotics will counteract that damage. Thus, it's not just what you add to your gut that creates health, but also what you remove. To create a hospitable environment, avoid products and activities that can harm the microbiome, such as unnecessary antibiotics, excessive sugar intake, pesticide-treated and genetically modified foods, chlorinated tap water, alcohol, cigarette smoking, poor sleep, inactivity, stress, and environmental toxins. Removing or reducing as many of these as possible prepares the gut for a productive seed-and-feed strategy, like tending the soil before planting.

Seeding the Gut

The first phase in the seed-and-feed strategy is to inoculate the gut with healthy bacteria. This was traditionally done with fermented foods, such as sauerkraut, kimchi, tempeh, miso, natto, yogurt, and kefir. And while these are still valuable parts of a healthy diet, we now also have the option of getting probiotics from a supplement—ideally a high-quality one with an adequate amount and variety of strains, including *Lactobacillus*, *Bifidobacterium*, and *Saccharomyces boulardii*. Both foods and supplements vary wildly in the number of colony-forming units (CFUs) and diversity of strains. Food and supplement labels will tell you the amount of live cultures (in CFUs) as well as the bacterial strains. While some people and certain conditions may benefit from a higher dosage, typical recommended dosages range from 1 to 20 billion CFUs per day, on an ongoing basis, for general gut health. With foods, choose products that retain high numbers of live cultures through the manufacturing process, such as ones which have not been heat-treated, or make your own fermented foods at home. Whether consuming probiotics through food, supplements, or a combination of both, diversity is important because it allows the microbiome to adapt more quickly to disruptions from the microbiome-harming factors we just discussed. In addition to consuming a variety of strains, microbiota diversity can also be increased through a diverse diet and by spending more time outside.

Feeding the Microbiota

When you seed the gut with beneficial bacteria, the best way to maintain a healthy population is by supplying adequate prebiotic fiber to feed them. Consume prebiotic-containing foods like onions, garlic, leeks, Jerusalem artichoke, oats, bananas, apples, and chicory root. To avoid digestive distress, proceed slowly when adding prebiotic foods into the diet. With this seed-and-feed strategy, gut health can improve in as little as a couple of weeks.

Supplements for Gut Health

Targeted supplementation can provide additional support along your path to optimal health. Supplements are discussed specifically within each section of this chapter (gut health, sleep, and stress) and guidance is provided at the end of the chapter for supplements to consider taking on trail as well as for post-trail recovery. It's important that you do your own research and work with your doctor when considering adding supplements to your wellness routine. They can interact with medications and have very real effects on the body. The information here is presented for educational purposes only and, ultimately, you must decide what's right for you. It's also important to buy quality supplements and follow the dosages on the labels unless instructed otherwise.

A healthy gut is a healthy body, and there are a few supplements that can help you repair the gut and maintain its health. In addition to a high-quality probiotic, other supplements that may enhance digestion, repair the gut lining, and support liver and gallbladder health include digestive bitters (dandelion, burdock, gentian, milk thistle, motherwort, goldenseal, and angelica), apple cider vinegar, digestive enzymes, L-glutamine, and herbs such as ginger root, dandelion root, peppermint leaf, and slippery elm bark.

PRIORITIZING SLEEP

Good sleep is critical to our physical and mental health, allowing the body to recover and repair each day. Deep sleep fortifies your immune system, balances hormones, supports healthy metabolism, increases energy, improves brain function, reduces stress, enhances muscle recovery, and boosts mood. It also reduces the risk for several diseases, including diabetes and heart disease, helps you make better decisions, improves motivation, and even reduces sugar cravings—all of which help you create resilient health, at home or on trail.

Most studies indicate that adults need seven to nine hours of sound sleep to reset their circadian rhythm and receive all the benefits associated with sleep. Unfortunately, most people either have trouble falling asleep or staying asleep. The effects of chronic sleep deprivation range from increased cancer risk and inflammation to cravings, reduced cognitive function, and irritability. In the busyness of our modern world, innumerable factors vie for your attention and distract you from deep sleep. Carving out time for sleep requires that you make it a priority, and preparation for a good night's rest begins as soon as you wake up. As you implement the sleep practices outlined in this section, keep in mind that it may take about a month to see consistent results. Hang in there. It's worth it. Sound sleep enables you to perform optimally and to create the health necessary to get outside and thrive on your adventures.

Supporting Deep Sleep

Human beings evolved with natural day and night cycles. These circadian rhythms regulate hormone production, such as cortisol and melatonin, which influence our sleep-wake cycles. Cortisol and melatonin oppose each other: cortisol naturally peaks within an hour of waking and then slowly declines throughout the day, allowing melatonin to rise and create deep sleep. When the natural rhythm of these hormones is disrupted, sleep disturbances result. Because both cortisol and melatonin are powerfully affected by light exposure, you can reset their natural rhythms by waking up at the same time each morning and exposing your eyes to outdoor light within an hour of sunrise. This sets the timer for melatonin to rise fourteen to sixteen hours later. If you can't get outside, sit near a window where natural light is pouring in. Sunlight is ideal, however, as it's significantly brighter than indoor light.

Habits you can implement during the day to support deeper sleep at night include avoiding daytime naps longer than twenty minutes, exercising for at least thirty minutes early in the day, and eating no later than three hours before bed. It's also helpful to avoid nicotine and alcohol near bedtime and set a caffeine curfew. It can take up to ten hours for caffeine to completely clear your system, so cutting yourself off by noon is optimal.

In addition to daytime habits, what you do in the hours leading up to sleep can have a

Heather Tip

On trail you will hear the term "hiker midnight" used to refer to 9:00 pm. Long-distance hikers rapidly adjust their circadian rhythms to match the sun cycle—waking up near sunrise and going to sleep around sunset. However, the ability to take electronics into the backcountry can make it tempting to stay awake in the tent watching a blue screen. This can lead to similar disruptions as at home. For me, the synchronization with the sun is part of why I feel incredibly healthy on the trail, so I avoid screen time in the tent.

dramatic effect on sleep latency and quality. Establishing a relaxing evening routine signals to your body that it's time to wind down. This could include taking an aromatherapy bath with Epsom salts and essential oils, reading fiction, writing in a journal, doing yin yoga, or listening to guided meditations. Your sleep will also benefit from avoiding bright lights and screens (TV, phone, iPad, etc.) for at least an hour before you plan to be asleep because the blue light from screens disrupts melatonin production, preventing you from sleeping as deeply. To reduce blue-light exposure after sunset, consider using blue-light blocking glasses and apps like f.lux. These habits are most effective when practiced consistently.

Create a Sleep Sanctuary

Deep sleep will be a challenge if your sleep environment is not calming. To ensure a restful night, make your bedroom your sleep sanctuary by cleaning up clutter, removing electronics, and reducing ambient noise and light. You may also benefit from using an eye mask, blackout curtains, or earplugs. Thermoregulation also impacts sleep: Studies have found that the ideal room temperature for sleep is 60 to 67 degrees Fahrenheit. Finally, invest in a comfortable mattress, pillows, and bedding. Choosing dust-mite resistant and nontoxic bedding options and also a quality air filter can greatly assist with reducing breathing issues that many people experience due to dust allergies and off-gassing of petroleum-based components.

Supplements for Sleep

If you're engaging in the lifestyle practices outlined in the preceding section and still struggling with sleep, you might consider a few thoughtfully chosen natural sleep aids. Always check with your doctor before taking any new supplement or herb, especially if you are pregnant, nursing, or taking any prescription medications.

One powerful sleep aid is magnesium, which can relax tense muscles, reduce pain, and calm the nervous system. There are many forms of magnesium: the ones commonly used for sleep are magnesium glycinate and magnesium threonate. Another popular sleep aid is the hormone melatonin, which works for some people but causes wakefulness in others and can be a hormone disruptor. L-theanine, the calming compound found in green tea, is another option. Lastly, nervines are a class of herbs that have traditionally been used to calm the nervous system and induce sound sleep. Examples include chamomile, passionflower, California poppy, hops, ashwagandha, and valerian. Herbs also come with caution, so it's important to do your own research or work with a qualified professional to determine what's best for you.

MINIMIZING STRESS

A few years after my post-PCT health issues, I was feeling better, but I wasn't fully recovered. Even though I had learned so much about nutrition, hormone health, and what the body truly needs to maintain long-term health, and I was consuming an anti-inflammatory diet, exercising enough (but not too much), and getting enough sleep most of the time, I still didn't feel 100 percent. I had lingering symptoms like brain fog, afternoon fatigue, and reduced endurance that indicated I wasn't back to my full potential. I felt like I was doing everything I was "supposed" to be doing to create optimal health, but I wasn't quite there. What else could there be?

During my research and educational training, I had often read about stress and the severe consequences it could have on nearly every aspect of health. I took in the information and filed it away for later because I didn't feel stressed, so I assumed I wasn't experiencing any of its effects. But the tricky thing about stress is that it feels different for each person. It doesn't always show up as the driver with road rage or the angry boss we envision as the caricature of someone who is "stressed." Sometimes it shows up as sadness, anger, a lack of motivation, or feeling overwhelmed, among other emotions. I didn't feel stressed, but I knew something was still getting in the way of my healing, so I figured it couldn't hurt to do as much as possible to address the potential stressors in my life. I spent a few weeks identifying and actively reducing the various stressors in my life, and eventually I did experience improvements in mental clarity and workout performance. Stress management is still the health practice that's most difficult for me to keep a handle on, but I now have no doubt that when I let it slip, my performance in every area of life also slips.

Stress has the potential to undermine any other positive changes you're making to your health. You can be eating well, taking supplements, and moving your body, but if you're stressed, you won't fully optimize your health and performance. Stress management may not seem relevant to preparing for a long hike, but it absolutely is if you want to perform at your peak!

We often think of stress as a feeling, but it's actually a physiological response that occurs when the body is met with physical, emotional, and mental challenges. When you encounter stress, whether real or perceived, the adrenal glands release the stress hormone cortisol into the bloodstream to make you focused and alert. Your heart rate increases and glucose is released to fuel your muscles so you can escape the danger. The immune system responds by producing inflammation. Once danger has passed, cortisol levels return to normal, insulin takes care of the extra blood sugar that was released, inflammation subsides, and all is well. At least, that's how it should work.

Historically, dangers for humans were short-lived. This is still true for most of the natural world: Imagine the classic example of the lion chasing the gazelle. The gazelle goes into the flight response, outruns the lion, and then goes back to grazing. In small amounts, stress can be a positive force, even life-saving, but in larger amounts, it becomes harmful to the body and mind. The problem occurs when the danger or perceived danger never stops. This is common in our modern world, where stress comes in many forms, from physical stress, such as overtraining, to emotional and psychological stress, such as concerns over finances and relationships, to the chemical stress of toxins in our environment. When we're constantly stressed, in addition to having extra cortisol in our bodies, we also pump out extra insulin which leads to insulin resistance, weight gain, and cravings for sugar, salt, and fat. Our productivity-focused culture encourages us to push too hard, take on too much, and believe that we can fit in everything. This is not how we're meant to live. Stress contributes to the development of all diseases and disorders, from increased susceptibility to the common cold to autoimmune disease, cardiovascular disease, metabolic syndrome, sleep disturbances, and systemic inflammation. For athletes, chronic stress results in slower recovery times, increased muscle fatigue, and lack of focus and motivation.

When considering the effects of stress on the body, it's important to consider the concept of allostatic load—that is, the wear and tear on the body from accumulated stressors. There's a certain amount of stress the body can adapt to no matter the source or type, but at a certain point, it can no longer cope and performance suffers. Imagine that each person has a "stress cup": Stress comes in a variety of forms, with each filling your stress cup a little more. Your body is capable of coping with stress at a certain rate, reducing the amount in your cup. If the stress being added to the cup exceeds your body's ability to adapt, your cup overflows. When that happens, you experience the deleterious effects of allostatic overload, including many of the common diseases of modern life.

Understanding the different forms of stress is key to identifying the sources in your life so that you can address them and reduce their effects. Sources of stress can be physical, chemical, or psychological: Physical stressors include injuries, overtraining, lack of sleep, and dietary triggers. Examples of chemical stressors are environmental pollutants and toxins in our personal care products, cleaning products, and sprayed onto our food. Emotional and psychological stressors are the ones we most commonly think of when we think about stress. These could include financial stress, an argument with a loved one, a divorce, being late to a meeting, and getting stuck in traffic. To reduce the likelihood of psychological stressors taking a toll on your health and performance, you can prevent them or mitigate them.

Preventing Stress

Ideally you prevent stress before it even happens. One technique to do this is to get better at saying no. Be honest with yourself about what you can reasonably take on, and don't be afraid to say no to more things, including commitments and social events that don't excite you.

Another method to reduce stress is to schedule must-do items on your calendar, as well as any additional time involved like driving to and from an event. This provides a more realistic picture of what you can commit to and what you can't.

An additional tactic to prevent the buildup of stress over the course of the day is to take more breaks. If your work environment permits, consider committing to three or four focused work blocks of 90 to 120 minutes each in your day. Reset for 15 to 20 minutes between blocks by getting away from your workstation. Go out for a short walk, snuggle your pet, drink water, breathe deeply, and allow yourself to rest for a moment.

Mitigating Stress

We can do our best to avoid stress, but we can't completely eliminate it from our lives. Therefore, it's important to have reliable practices that help you manage it more effectively. Practice these techniques consistently to see results, and in doing so, you can shift how you experience the world. You'll be able to regulate your cortisol production (which will help you sleep better), balance body weight, have more energy, improve your endurance, and stay more present in your life so you can truly enjoy it. Plus, when you keep your stress in check, you'll be able to train harder and hike longer.

> *As a natural-born worrier, stress has been a part of my life since birth. Just like Katie, I frequently underestimated the amount of stress in my life because I didn't "feel" stressed. However, when I began my athletic journey outside of backpacking (ultra-marathon running), I began to notice indicators of stress taking its toll on my health. Integrating stress-reducing activities into my life such as yoga and meditation has been instrumental in lowering my overall stress. Chapter 8 covers mental preparation techniques for the trail, and all of these can be used prior to and post hike as part of daily stress management.*

Reframing Stressful Events

The intensity of our response to a particular stressor depends largely on perception, and so we can change our stress response by changing our perception of the event. In psychology, this is called reframing. This technique can be used in the moment to shift how you perceive an event and therefore shift your body out of a stress response.

By cultivating an intentional reaction to events we perceive as threatening, we can gain a greater sense of control and lessen the physiological impacts of stress. Stress largely develops from a sense of lack of control, and reframing helps you gain a little of that control back. Keep in mind that reframing depends entirely on your ability to stay present when you're experiencing stress. Reframing is a habit, and the more you practice, the more you rewire your brain and the easier it becomes.

To reframe stress, try the following techniques developed by Chris Kresser, a leading functional medicine clinician:

- **Question your thoughts.** Recognize that you don't have to believe your thoughts. Question whether they are true or just a perception.
- **Interpret a threat as a challenge.** Ask yourself if you can find an opportunity in the event. For example, a health diagnosis may be a better opportunity to care for yourself.
- **Expand your time horizon.** Consider how much the event actually matters and whether or not you will be concerned about it in a month, a year, or a decade.
- **Increase your sense of control.** It's your sense of control rather than actually being in control that impacts how you perceive stress. Focus on the things that are under your control and do your best to find creative solutions.

Relaxation Techniques for Acute Stress

Acute stress is the type that comes on quickly and unexpectedly, throwing you off-balance

BREATHWORK TECHNIQUES	
TECHNIQUE	**INSTRUCTIONS**
4-7-8 BREATHING	Sit with your back straight. Place the tip of your tongue behind your upper front teeth. Inhale through the nose for 4 counts, hold breath for 7 counts, exhale through the mouth for 8 counts. Repeat 3 times.
BOX BREATHING	Sitting comfortably, exhale all air. Breathe in through the nose for 4 counts, hold for 4 counts, exhale through the mouth for 4 counts, hold at "empty" for 4 counts. Repeat 3 times.
ALTERNATE NOSTRIL BREATHING	Sit up straight in a comfortable seat. Close your eyes and inhale and exhale deeply. Softly close your right nostril with your right thumb, inhaling through the left nostril. Close your left nostril with your ring finger so that both nostrils are closed for a moment, then open your right nostril and exhale slowly. Inhale through your right nostril, hold both nostrils closed for a moment, then open your left nostril and exhale slowly. Repeat 5 to 10 times.
2:1 BREATHING	Sitting or lying comfortably, inhale deeply through the nose to a moderate mental count, then exhale through the mouth for twice that count (double the duration). Repeat as many times as you'd like.

momentarily. This could include an argument with someone in your life or an exam for which you don't feel adequately prepared. Though it doesn't last long, it triggers your body's stress response, and you can reverse it with quick relaxation techniques. One powerful technique for acute stress is to use breathing exercises. These are great because they can be done anywhere and can shift you back into a relaxed state in minutes. See the breathwork chart above for more details.

Mindfulness practices, which ground you in your body in the present moment, are also effective for on-the-spot stress reduction. The simplest way to practice mindfulness is to notice what you're sensing in a given moment: the sights, sounds, and smells that ordinarily slip by without reaching your conscious awareness. There are also many excellent apps that can guide you to connect with your breath and your body. See Additional Resources for suggestions.

Tips for Coping with Chronic Stress
If the stress response is chronically triggered and the body is not brought back to a relaxed state before the next wave of stress hits, the body can stay triggered indefinitely. This chronic stress slowly breaks the body down and can lead to the health issues discussed earlier. Managing this type of stress often requires a combined approach of using the acute stress-relief practices outlined above along with long-term stress-relief habits such as regular exercise, maintaining a healthy diet, spending time in nature, engaging in hobbies, and listening to music. Make your mindfulness and meditation practices into long-term habits to get the best results. Additionally, cultivating deep relationships and spending time with people you love releases oxytocin, which directly combats stress. On a long-distance hike, there will be many times when you need to remain calm during the storm (literally and figuratively!). Learning how to identify and mitigate stress is essential.

Adrenal Health for Adventurers
Many individuals who are drawn to endurance sports are driven, ambitious people. That type of intensity is not just how they approach sport, it's how they approach life. While drive, determination, and hard work are invaluable to achievement, these same tendencies often push

high achievers beyond what is reasonable and healthy. When you push too hard for too long, the effects of chronic stress on the body lead to a condition called hypothalamic-pituitary-adrenal (HPA) axis dysregulation. The HPA axis is the body's main stress-response system. Dysfunction affects systems throughout the body, including the thyroid and metabolism, immune function, brain function, and hormone production. HPA axis dysregulation can present differently for each person. According to integrative physician Dr. Aviva Romm, the most common signs that you're in adrenal overdrive include trouble falling asleep even though you're tired and not feeling rested when you wake; getting irritable more quickly than normal; cravings for sugar, fat, and salt; afternoon fatigue; weight gain around your middle; feeling anxious or blue; getting sick more often; fertility problems; reduced libido; impaired memory and focus; and digestive system distress.

HPA axis dysregulation exists on a spectrum ranging from adrenal overdrive to burnout to exhaustion. As mentioned, chronic stress drives HPA axis dysregulation, and that stress can come from any of the sources outlined earlier. For the long-distance hiker, this may include worrying that you're not going to successfully finish the trail, that you'll run out of money, or that you won't find a job when you get home. Physical stressors like walking 20-plus miles daily, sleeping poorly, and having a nutrient-deficient diet all contribute to the overall stress on the body. Furthermore, chronically under-eating and over-exercising, which are common on a long hike, create additional stress on the body. This can result in impaired thyroid function, reduced sex hormones, and increased cortisol while your body tries to meet the demands of these stressors. Left unchecked, this process can culminate in HPA axis dysregulation.

Keep in mind that it may not be obvious that you're overstressing your body, especially if you're on a long backpacking trip, where fatigue is an inevitable part of the activity. Returning to the concept of allostatic load, the body can adapt up until a certain threshold. Reducing any stressors you have control over, such as diet and sleep, can help your body keep up with the demands. In some cases, you may not notice that you've overtaxed your adrenals until after your hike. The sooner you notice symptoms however, the better, as you can then begin to ease up, allow your body to repair itself, and get back to feeling good more quickly. While hiking the PCT, I felt great for the majority of my hike. I didn't experience any injuries or illnesses. It wasn't until I returned home, went through significant emotional stress, and tried to start training for my next ultramarathon that I discovered my stamina was completely gone. Additional symptoms, such as lethargy, muscle fatigue, and digestive distress indicated to me that my adrenals were struggling. Looking back, there were indications toward the end of my hike that my body needed rest. However,

Heather Tip

In the year leading up to my 2013 PCT fastest known time (FKT), I experienced a series of health issues, including chronic injury and multiple deficiencies. Due to my stubborn, driven, and ambitious nature, I went on my hike anyway. Although I was successful, the incredible stress on my body took a very long time to recover from. In retrospect, I should have continued working with my health-care providers to solve the underlying issue that turned out to be a food intolerance. Had I discovered this prior to setting out, I could have taken the time to heal my body through supplementation and removal of the food stressor, which would have made me stronger on trail. The combined stress of my physical body, the improper fueling, and the rigors of hiking 45-plus miles per day nearly destroyed my health. Do not discount the importance of building a resilient body prior to starting your hike!

I ignored them and tried to keep training as soon as I returned home, even though I was dealing with emotional stress as well. My body's messages became louder. I finally heeded the warnings, but it took several months to reverse the damage.

You can confirm HPA axis dysregulation by taking a cortisol test with your doctor, but if you're experiencing any of these symptoms, you don't need to wait for a test to begin nourishing your adrenals. This book covers several strategies to help you do that. The first is to remove inflammatory triggers from your diet and regulate your blood sugar. Caffeine can be a stressor, so eliminating or reducing it supports adrenal health. Maintaining good sleep habits is also critical. Review the list of emotional, physical, and environmental stressors listed earlier and reflect on how you can reduce or eliminate them.

Above all, listen to your body. It's always giving you signals. Be cognizant of how you feel after a workout. After my own forays into adrenal overdrive, I no longer ignore tiredness, fatigue, or soreness while training. Exercise should energize you, not drain you. Training with long distances is helpful, but don't deplete yourself and end your hike before you even begin. Finding the right training plan for you is essential; turn to chapter 7 for more on this topic.

Supplements for Stress

Even when you're eating a healthy diet, you can run low on key nutrients, and stress depletes them even faster. Magnesium, B-vitamins, vitamin D, and L-theanine are particularly supportive during times of increased stress. Additionally, adaptogenic herbs such as ashwagandha, eleuthero root, or *Rhodiola rosea* have a long history of traditional use in various cultures as well as a growing body of scientific research indicating their ability to regulate stress response via the HPA axis.

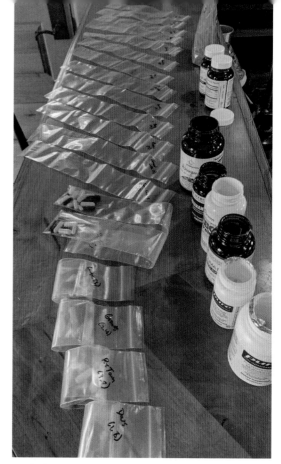

Portioning supplements for resupply boxes

SPENDING MORE TIME OUTSIDE

If you're reading this book, you're probably already intuitively aware of how nature immersion improves physical and mental health. American biologist E. O. Wilson popularized the concept of biophilia—love of life and the living world—in 1984 based on his belief that because humans evolved in nature, we have a biological need to connect with it. There's now research to confirm this.

Although humans have an innate connection to the earth, we have increasingly become an urban species, spending the majority of our time indoors. According to research in the book *Forest Bathing* by Dr. Qing Li, this has resulted in anxiety, headaches, depression, mental fatigue, eye strain, insomnia, frustration, irritability, and reduced quality of life. A growing body of data suggests that connection to nature can improve cardiovascular and metabolic health, concentration and memory, pain thresholds, energy, and immune function. Of particular importance is the effect that nature immersion has on the nervous system. Research indicates that the practice of walking in the forest lowers the stress hormones cortisol and adrenaline, suppresses the sympathetic nervous system, enhances the parasympathetic nervous system, lowers blood pressure, and increases heart-rate variability. Our "affinity for the natural world is fundamental to our health. [It's] as vital to our well-being as regular exercise and a healthy diet. Just as our health improves when we are in it, so our health suffers when we are divorced from it," Qing writes. Forest bathing—just walking or spending time in the forest—is one more tool you can use to fight chronic inflammation and optimize health.

And a study published in *Nature*, which included twenty thousand participants, indicated that 120 minutes per week in the outdoors, whether that's an urban park or a more remote setting, is significantly associated with good health and a sense of well-being. Results applied across different ethnic groups, socioeconomic classes, genders, and levels of baseline health. This is one more reason to prioritize outdoor training sessions as you're preparing for your next adventure!

> **Heather Tip**
>
> *As someone with a compromised gut biome and poor absorption resulting from a food intolerance, supplements have been crucial to my health while on trail. Under the guidance of my health-care provider, I developed a list of vitamins, minerals, and adaptogens that—combined with a revamped healthy-food strategy—support me during my long-distance hikes.*

SUPPLEMENTS AND HERBS

Throughout this chapter, I have discussed specific supplements that may enhance your health as you prepare for the trail. You may be wondering if it's worth the extra pack weight to carry supplements on trail as well. I encourage a "food first" approach. However, due to decreased availability of fresh foods on trail as well as the increased rate of nutrient depletion during heavy exercise, supplements can be a good form of nutritional insurance. With the extreme physical demands placed on the body during a long-distance hike, supplementation can support improved energy and endurance, enhanced immune function, faster recovery, and reduced illness and fatigue. I find that they are worth the weight and expense. The following is not an exhaustive list of "performance" supplements, but contains a handful of well-researched options specifically geared toward hikers.

Taking supplements regularly on trail requires you to either carry the whole bottle or to send them to yourself in resupply boxes. When choosing supplements for the trail, select shelf-stable options (most are, but check probiotics and fish oil, in particular) since you won't have access to regular refrigeration. If sending them in resupply boxes, consult your resupply spreadsheet and divvy up the supplements into baggies corresponding to the number of days of food in each box. Calculate accordingly if there are certain locations where you won't be sending a box.

High-Quality Multivitamin

A high-quality multivitamin is beneficial in helping you avoid micronutrient deficiencies you may incur due to the lack of fresh foods on trail. The micronutrients found in a good multivitamin play an important role in energy production, hemoglobin synthesis, maintenance of bone health, adequate immune function, and protection of the body against oxidative damage. Additionally, they assist with synthesis and repair of muscle tissue.

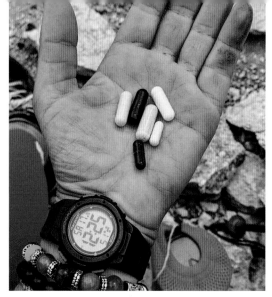

Supplements can be part of a daily wellness routine on trail.

Spore-Based Probiotics

On top of promoting good gut health, probiotics have a host of other benefits, including boosting the immune system, supporting brain function, and enhancing mineral absorption. These healthy gut bacteria can even contribute to hormone balance and the production of certain neurotransmitters. There are many types of probiotic supplements to choose from. On trail, I use a spore-based probiotic because it's more shelf-stable than others. Additionally, certain spore-based probiotics have been shown to heal a condition known as leaky gut (intestinal hyperpermeability) by closing tight junctions between colonocytes, increasing the thickness of intestinal mucosa, and upregulating the body's natural defense against infections. This supplement may be helpful for hikers who are consuming little-to-no probiotic-rich foods and eating a less-than-ideal diet.

Krill Oil

Krill oil has been studied for its positive effects on brain and heart health and for keeping overall inflammation low. Most modern diets tend to be high in inflammatory omega-6 fats and low in anti-inflammatory omega-3 fats. Consuming krill oil, which is a rich source of omega-3 fat, helps you get closer to an optimal ratio of omega-6 to omega-3 in the diet. Krill oil is preferable to fish oil because it includes astaxanthin, a powerful antioxidant that protects the fragile fats from oxidizing, which can make them both ineffective and damaging to the body. Astaxanthin also serves as internal sunscreen by protecting the skin from damage caused by UV exposure. Heat, air, and light degrade oils, so how you store your krill oil is important: Use capsules rather than liquid, and keep them in a plastic bag in the middle of your pack, where temperatures are cooler and more stable.

Curcumin Turmeric

Turmeric, a root in the ginger family, is a major source of curcumin, a polyphenol that has powerful antioxidant and anti-inflammatory effects. According to a 2017 research review of curcumin's effects on human health, "It aids in the management of oxidative and inflammatory conditions, metabolic syndrome, arthritis, anxiety, and hyperlipidemia. It may also help in the management of exercise-induced inflammation and muscle soreness, thus enhancing recovery and subsequent performance in active people." Many curcumin supplements contain piperine, which increases the bioavailability of the curcumin by 2000 percent. If your supplement does not contain piperine, consuming black pepper with your turmeric can increase bioavailability.

Heather Tip

Early on in my hiking career, I noticed a frequent and insatiable craving for orange juice. Every time I reached town, I would buy and drink an entire jug! Eventually I surmised (after an assessment of my standard hiking-food nutrition labels) that I was severely deficient in dietary vitamin C. In the next town I bought some vitamin C supplements and never had a citrus craving again. Don't underestimate your body's ability to tell you what it needs.

Magnesium

Nearly half of all Americans are deficient in magnesium, which is required for more than three hundred biochemical reactions in the body. It's important for several functions, including muscle function and heartbeat, immunity, nerve cell function, energy production, and strong bones. There are many forms of magnesium to choose from: For sound sleep, magnesium glycinate and threonate are most effective. For general magnesium deficiency and a highly bioavailable form, magnesium glycinate is helpful. My protocol is to take magnesium powder dissolved in a small amount of liquid before bed to relax muscles, aid in recovery, and promote sound sleep. Magnesium right before sleep can give some people vivid (and sometimes sleep-disturbing) dreams. Experiment with the timing of taking magnesium before bed (up to several hours prior) to find the right time frame for your body.

Vitamin C

Vitamin C is critical for many functions in the body, including healthy immune function, wound healing, collagen production, body tissue repair, and the proper functioning of the adrenal glands. If you're taking a multivitamin, that may be adequate. However, given the lack of fresh fruits and veggies in the standard hiker diet coupled with the specific benefits vitamin C offers backpackers, I ensure I'm consuming enough by using vitamin C drink packets, which serve as a flavor enhancer for my water in addition to a multivitamin. The daily recommended amount of vitamin C is 60 to 95 milligrams, though thru-hikers' needs are likely above normal. It's unlikely that too much vitamin C is harmful, though doses above 2000 milligrams per day may cause diarrhea, nausea, and cramping.

Adaptogens for Hikers

As mentioned in the section on stress, adaptogens are a class of medicinal herbs and mushrooms that increase the ability of an organism to react to and resist stressors. Each adaptogen influences the body in a slightly different way. Though they have a long history of use in Ayurvedic and Chinese medicine, most herbs are still not well studied, unfortunately, so much of what we know is based on traditional use. Adaptogens that may enhance physical performance on trail include *Cordyceps* mushroom to boost stamina, *Rhodiola rosea* to reduce fatigue, *Schisandra* berry to improve endurance, and ashwagandha to improve aerobic capacity and time to exhaustion. Additionally, *Panax* ginseng has been found to enhance endurance by increasing aerobic capacity and reducing lactate production. On top of these, I also include natural anti-inflammatories like ginger, cinnamon, garlic, and turmeric in my food when possible.

Post-Trail Supplements and Herbs

Even the most well-trained hiker who adheres to the recommendations in this book will endure physical wear and tear on the body during a multi-month hike. In addition to providing your body with adequate rest after a backcountry adventure, you may wish to consider specific supplements to support your body in recovery and repair. For example, omega-3 fats from cold-water fish and curcumin from turmeric can reduce the inflammatory effects from months of hiking, and adaptogen and nervine herbs may be beneficial in helping the body recover more quickly from the stressors of a long-distance hike. Probiotics can support a backpacker by helping to restore gut health after weeks or months of relying on mostly shelf-stable food. A healthy microbiome is important for many functions in the body, including regulating inflammation, digesting food, and synthesizing vitamins, and it even plays a role in mood, which means that probiotics could be beneficial for hikers dealing with post-trail blues. For more on post-trail reintegration, see chapter 9.

6

PERFORMANCE NUTRITION & BACKCOUNTRY MEAL PLANNING

BY *Katie*

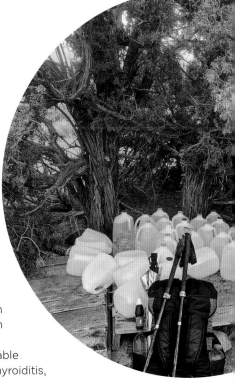

The level of exhaustion that washed over me when I finished thru-hiking the PCT was beyond anything I'd ever experienced. After walking nearly 2700 miles from Mexico to Canada, I was not the beacon of health I'd imagined I would be when I returned home to North Carolina. I experienced bone-deep fatigue, yet I couldn't sleep. My hands and feet were constantly cold, my hair was falling out in clumps, and I was battling depression. This all left me feeling uncertain about what was going on with my health and worried about what the future held for me as an outdoor endurance athlete.

Many months later, I discovered that my seemingly inexplicable symptoms were due to adrenal exhaustion and Hashimoto's thyroiditis, an autoimmune condition. I knew I wanted to try diet and lifestyle interventions to heal my body before turning to pharmaceuticals, so I designed a protocol that I hoped would allow me to return to the active outdoor lifestyle that I had built my identity around. I created this protocol over the course of months, after a great deal of reading, research, testing, and close work with a functional medicine practitioner (a health-care professional who focuses on identifying and addressing the underlying root causes of dysfunction). Improvements over the following months and years enabled me to regain my health, start running again, and eventually hike thousands more miles.

The nutrition principles I used to improve my own health, which are backed by research and years of traditional use, make up the foundation of the anti-inflammatory eating framework you'll find within the section on pre-trail nutrition in this chapter. Anti-inflammatory eating is not a "diet" per se, in that it's not about dogma, rules, and restriction. Rather it's an approach to eating that prioritizes nutrient-dense whole foods and the reduction of inflammation throughout the body. The principles of anti-inflammatory eating are straightforward, and you need not be suffering from a health condition to benefit from implementing them. This approach to nutrition can help you feel great regardless of the style of eating you follow and whether you have dietary restrictions or not. My personal journey has run the gamut from vegan to vegetarianism, keto to paleo. I now follow a flexible, personalized approach to nutrition that evolves as I do. This chapter provides the tools to determine what works best for you at home and as your needs change throughout your life.

This chapter also includes a section about how to fuel your body for performance once you're on trail. After I'd become healthy enough to hike again, my goal was to transition my anti-inflammatory diet to the trail as seamlessly as possible so that I could retain optimal well-being on my hikes. A long-distance hike demands a lot of the body, and I knew my nutrition needed to be on point if I wanted to avoid being forced off trail early due to depletion. As a lifelong athlete and student of biology, the direct correlation between nutrition and performance was clear to me: My on-trail nutrition needed to fuel ten or more hours daily of moderate-intensity exercise for months on end. The standard ramen and Snickers thru-hiker diet wasn't going to cut it for me. I needed optimal fuel.

Not only does food quality affect on-trail performance, hikers must also take into consideration the macronutrients that are best suited for long-distance hiking and the need for lightweight, shelf-stable fare. The on-trail nutrition

Heather Tip

Much like Katie, I've seen a direct correlation between my athletic performance on trail and my diet. I also experimented with many different styles of eating (vegan, vegetarian, paleo, etc.) in an attempt to correct what I intrinsically knew was a food sensitivity. I set the PCT FKT in 2013 while ingesting tons of crackers, cookies, tortillas, etc., but I finished that hike emaciated, and I knew that it would take a very long time to heal. Eventually I discovered the underlying issue: gluten intolerance. For many years, and during one of the hardest physical endeavors of my life, I'd been poisoning my body with the food I was eating. ● Although my case, like Katie's, is extreme, it demonstrates the connection between input and output very concretely. Once I finally had a diagnosis, I overhauled my off-trail diet and healed. When I set out on the AT to set an FKT just a year later, my on-trail nutrition followed the guidelines in this book and was completely free of gluten. My performance increase was significant, as was my body's ability to recover and heal from the hike.

section of this chapter outlines an approach for the long-distance hiker who is concerned with both weight savings and performance.

PRE-HIKE NUTRITION

Improving your nutrition in the months leading up to your hike can be instrumental in achieving higher mileage days, faster recovery, better stamina, and fewer injuries on the trail. This section provides strategies to help you create optimal health so you can build the most resilient body possible before embarking on your adventure. A backpacking trip, whether it's a few days or a few months, is rigorous. Hiking all day with a backpack on, sometimes in extreme weather, demands a lot from the body, which in turn depletes nutrient reserves more quickly. As discussed in the previous chapter, a depleted body is more likely to succumb to injury, illness, and fatigue, all of which can cause you to abandon your hike early.

Starting off in optimal health, with nutrient reserves topped off, is particularly important for backpackers, who have reduced access to nutrient-dense foods like fresh fruits and vegetables once they hit the trail. Fresh foods contain high levels of antioxidants, which combat the free-radical damage induced by heavy physical demands. The longer your backpacking trip, the greater the likelihood you will become depleted, so improving your pre-trip nutrition sets you up for greater success once you hit the trail.

Biochemical Individuality

Before getting into the specifics of how to eat for optimal health and performance, let's explore the concept of biochemical individuality, because it affects every aspect of your health. Biochemical individuality, or bio-individuality, as coined by biochemist Dr. Roger Williams in 1956, refers to the idea that we are all genetically and biochemically unique,

and therefore, dietary and other needs must be modified from one person to the next. While all human bodies are made up of the same organs and processes, there are fluctuations in your body's biochemistry that are unique to you. This individuality is due to your genetics, the diversity of your microbiome, your health history, and your levels of inflammation. These differences influence how we process both macro- and micronutrients. It explains, at least in part, why two people can respond differently to the same exact meal—why your hiking partner feels great eating keto, while the same diet leaves you feeling sluggish and foggy.

As such, bio-individuality makes clear the limitations inherent in universal dietary guidelines. It's the reason why there is no single "best" diet for everyone. That said, there are some universal nutrition principles—covered next—that benefit nearly everyone. After that, we discuss how to further customize your diet for your unique body. Ultimately, you know your body best, and your internal guidance should be the backdrop against which you evaluate the information provided here.

Anti-Inflammatory Eating

In chapter 5, we covered the role of inflammation in peak performance. We looked at nondietary sources of inflammation as well as prevention and mitigation strategies. This chapter outlines dietary sources of inflammation and how that inflammation impacts the aspiring backpacker. Consider this: any food you put into your body is either fueling the fire of inflammation or fighting it. Though food insecurity and access are real issues that need to be addressed, many of us are fortunate enough to control what we eat each day, and we can begin to lower inflammation starting with our next meal. The following anti-inflammatory dietary practices are present in the longest-lived and healthiest populations worldwide.

Limiting Inflammatory Foods

The first step in reducing systemic inflammation is to limit or remove the foods that are contributing factors. These are generally the highly processed ones, such as refined carbohydrates, processed seed and vegetable oils, artificial sweeteners, trans fats, and alcohol. It's not that the world's longest-lived populations never enjoy treats, but generally those indulgences are antioxidant-rich pleasures like fruit, nuts, herbal teas, wine, and coffee—not donuts and Cheetos.

Aiming for 80 Percent Whole Foods

Focus on whole foods over packaged or processed foods. This includes a variety of colorful fruits and vegetables, grass-fed meats, eggs, legumes, and raw nuts and seeds. Herbs, spices, and healthy fats—such as olive oil, coconut oil, walnut oil, and avocado oil—are also included in this category. By prioritizing foods in their whole form, you prioritize nutrient density. This provides the body with the vitamins and minerals it needs to repair and regenerate. What's more, the water and fiber in whole foods is satiating and naturally regulates your appetite.

Think of food as being on a spectrum, with whole, minimally refined foods at one end and highly processed and manipulated food at the opposite end. You will invariably need to eat food from the space in between those two extremes. When you do, you may need to choose foods that are packaged and processed, but ideally they are composed of only a few real food ingredients that you can recognize and pronounce. For example, if you purchase a meal replacement bar, which is clearly a processed food to some degree, look for an option that is made from a handful of whole food ingredients, such as dried fruit and nuts rather than the one that contains dozens of ingredients you don't recognize. By limiting foods from the highly processed end of the continuum, you reduce your intake of inflammatory food triggers, such as excess sugar, high-fructose corn syrup, trans fats, preservatives, and food colorings.

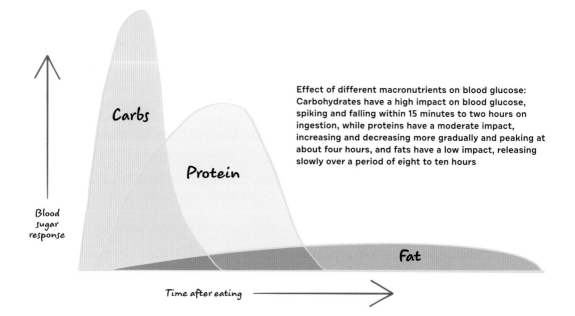

Carbs

Protein

Fat

Blood sugar response

Time after eating

Effect of different macronutrients on blood glucose: Carbohydrates have a high impact on blood glucose, spiking and falling within 15 minutes to two hours on ingestion, while proteins have a moderate impact, increasing and decreasing more gradually and peaking at about four hours, and fats have a low impact, releasing slowly over a period of eight to ten hours

Eating a Plant-Rich Diet

Plants are a rich source of micronutrients, the vitamins and minerals that are necessary for energy production, immune function, fluid balance, bone health, and much more. Antioxidants in plant foods help you to combat the free-radical damage and oxidative stress that is the result of the myriad stressors you encounter every day. Plants are also an important source of fiber. Fiber helps you eliminate waste properly and is essential for the health of your microbiome, and as we've mentioned, the microbiome affects virtually every aspect of health, including immune function, digestion, mood, and brain health. A diet rich in plants is a cornerstone of anti-inflammatory eating!

Stabilizing Blood Sugar with a Balance of Macronutrients

If you've had the experience of getting "hangry" between meals, you've experienced the effects of blood-sugar swings. Glucose levels in the bloodstream, a.k.a. blood-sugar levels, naturally vary throughout the day. Large spikes and drops, however, result in energy crashes, cravings, brain fog, anxiety, and hormone fluctuations that can drive inflammation, weight gain, and other challenges. The goal, then, is to prevent massive fluctuations. The macronutrients with which you fuel your body play a major role in blood-sugar variations. Macronutrients include carbohydrates, fats, and protein: they make up all of the food that you eat, and they're responsible for creating energy in your body, among other functions.

Carbohydrates

Carbohydrates are either simple or complex, and your digestive system breaks them down into glucose to provide energy. Simple carbohydrates are found naturally in foods like fruit and milk, as well as in processed foods like baked goods, soda, and table sugar. They are absorbed quickly and provide quick bursts of energy. Complex carbohydrates are found in vegetables, whole grains, and legumes. They're higher in fiber and are digested more slowly.

Protein

Protein is essential for every cell in the body. It is necessary for the enzymes that facilitate your metabolism, for the production of neurotransmitters that affect sleep and mood, and for muscle repair and growth. It's the most satiating macronutrient and is important for balancing blood sugar. Composed of chains of amino acids, proteins are either complete or incomplete. Complete proteins contain all the amino acids needed by the body. Examples include fish, meat, and milk. Incomplete protein sources lack one or more of the nine essential amino acids, which are the amino acids that can't be produced by the body. Beans, nuts, and tofu are examples. Incomplete sources can be consumed together to create a complete protein.

Fat

Fat provides energy, maintains cell membranes, protects organs, and is essential for proper brain function and hormone production. Fats are made up of fatty acids, which can be saturated or unsaturated. Saturated fats are found in animal products like beef, pork, and dairy, as well as plant foods, like coconut oil and cocoa butter. Unsaturated fats are either monounsaturated or polyunsaturated. Examples include olive oil, avocados, vegetable oils, and most nuts.

Each macronutrient is metabolized differently. Carbohydrates cause blood glucose levels to rise, which causes the pancreas to produce insulin. Insulin takes glucose from the bloodstream and shuttles it into cells for energy or storage. When large amounts of simple

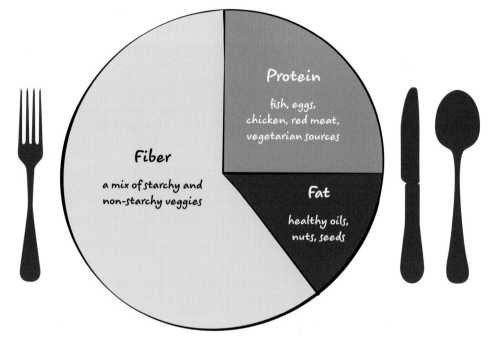

Template for a blood-sugar–balanced meal

carbohydrates are consumed, the body rapidly produces insulin in an attempt to keep up. This causes blood glucose levels to drop quickly, resulting in hypoglycemia, also known as a sugar crash. Fats and proteins, however, release energy into the bloodstream at a slower rate. This results in more sustained and lasting energy. Eating fiber-containing meals also blunts the insulin response, creating the same slow-burn effect.

To better understand this concept, think of feeding a fire. Simple carbohydrates are like kindling, which burns hot and fast. Fats and protein, on the other hand, are the logs, which burn slow and steady. This is a simplified explanation but is sufficient for our purposes. To achieve balanced blood sugar and more steady energy levels, include fat, protein, and fiber with each meal or snack.

Finding What Works for You

If you followed the tips for anti-inflammatory eating outlined in the preceding section and went no further with your dietary strategy, you would already be well on your way to vibrant health. For those who wish to dive deeper into customizing their nutrition strategy by looking at calorie and macronutrient intakes, determining your daily energy (calorie) target can help you achieve specific body-composition goals, and experimenting with different macronutrient ratios will allow you to determine what helps you feel and perform best. This information will be useful for optimizing your pre-trip nutrition as well as when it comes to planning your backpacking meals.

You can begin to build your nutrition strategy by tracking calories and macronutrients, but remember the concept of bio-individuality: the amount of calories you require daily and the macronutrient ratios you feel best eating is unique to you.

Estimating Your Target Energy Intake

A calorie is simply the amount of energy required to raise one liter of water by one degree centigrade in a laboratory setting; this fact alone doesn't take into account the complexity of your endocrine system, your metabolism, your microbiome, or even the quality of the food you're eating—all of which can influence what happens to calories in your body and how the food you eat affects your health. Keep in mind that food is information for the body, and you're affecting your hormones and mitochondria by what you eat. So estimating your daily calorie requirements can be a helpful starting point, but proper nutrition is about more than just calories.

To determine your daily calorie needs, you can use a free basal metabolic rate (BMR) and Harris-Benedict equation calculator on the internet (see Additional Resources). These take into account your age, gender, height, weight, and activity level to provide an estimate of the amount of calories you require to maintain body weight at your projected activity level.

Determining Ideal Macronutrient Ranges

Macronutrient ratios are more complex. Nutrition science is always evolving, and you'll find a lot of information on "ideal" ratios for different populations and activities. For instance, the USDA recommends that adults get 45 to 65 percent of their daily calories from carbohydrates. Meanwhile, there's a growing body of research suggesting the metabolic benefits of reduced-carbohydrate diets. Ultimately, like many health recommendations, what's ideal for you depends on several factors, many of which are unique to you. You can begin with a baseline and then use strategic self-experimentation to refine. Keep in mind that your ideal macronutrient ratios will also change depending on the type and intensity of physical activity you're engaging in.

To determine your baseline macronutrient numbers, begin with your protein number. The American College of Sports Medicine recommends 0.55 to 0.90 grams of protein per pound of body weight per day for athletes, depending on training. Strength-training athletes will be on the higher end, while endurance athletes, such as long-distance hikers, will be on the lower end of that range. To determine what percentage of your target daily calorie intake protein represents, multiply your protein target (in grams) by four (the number of calories per gram of protein), then divide that number by your total daily calories. Multiply the result by 100 to get a percentage.

Percent of daily calories from protein = [(target amount of protein (grams) × 4) ÷ target amount of calories] × 100

Next, you'll calculate your target carbohydrate and fat percentages. Some individuals feel better on higher-carbohydrate and lower-fat diets,

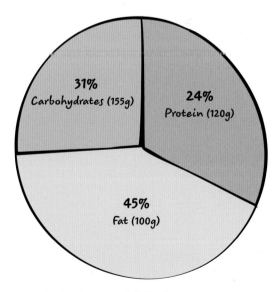

Example of daily macronutrient ratios

while others feel better on lower-carbohydrate and higher-fat diets. Once you know your protein percentage, subtract that number from 100 and divide the remainder of the calories between fat and carbohydrates to come up with a percentage for each. For reference, the USDA recommended fat intake for healthy adults is 20 to 25 percent of total calories. This does not, however, mean that's the appropriate percentage for you.

Based on your calculations, settle on a macronutrient percentage of fat, carbohydrate, and protein to start with. Track your intake and stick to those ratios for two weeks to see how you feel. You can track your intake by hand or use an app, which I find much easier (see Additional Resources). Monitor energy levels, moods,

cravings, and any weight changes. After two weeks, adjust if necessary. You may also want to consider working with a nutrition coach to support you through this process.

Keep in mind that the human body is not a machine, so these numbers are simply intended to provide a starting point. The best feedback will come from paying attention to your body. The goal is not to continue tracking forever but to gain a better understanding of the function of each macronutrient in your body, which macronutrient ratios leave you feeling your best, and what level of calorie intake allows you to meet your goals. After a month or two, you will likely have a good idea of your sweet spot. From there, rely on internal cues, such as appetite and hunger and fullness, to guide your choices.

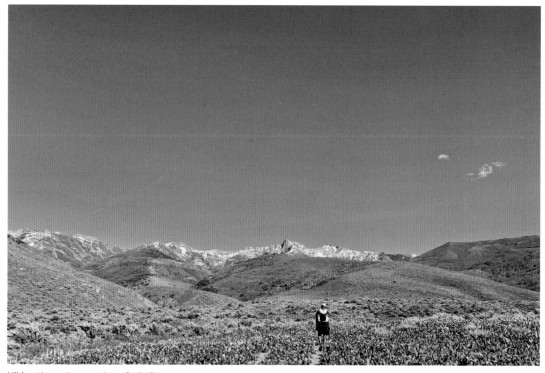

Hiking through a meadow of wildflowers on the way up to the Ruby Crest in Nevada

Mindful Eating Practices

The anti-inflammatory eating framework covers *what* to eat, but just as important for optimal health is *how* you eat. The state you are in when you sit down to a meal plays an important role in digestion, nutrient absorption, portion control, and inflammation. In our on-the-go culture, it's not uncommon to eat in a distracted, stressed state, often on the way from one place to the next.

The autonomic nervous system has two branches: sympathetic, which is often called "fight or flight," and parasympathetic, which is often called "rest and digest." In a stressed, sympathetic-dominant state, blood is shunted from the digestive system to the muscles to enable rapid escape from danger. In contrast, in a relaxed, parasympathetic-dominant state, blood is directed to the digestive system so that the body can properly digest, assimilate, absorb, and eliminate the ingested food.

To shift into a parasympathetic state before your next meal, slow down. Sit down, ideally at a table instead of in your car or in front of a screen. Take ten deep breaths and pause for a moment of gratitude before taking your first bite. Healthy digestion begins in the mind before food even enters the mouth. The sight and smell of food allow the salivary glands to begin producing the enzymes necessary to initiate the breakdown of food. Give yourself a moment to savor the sensory experience of a meal before you begin eating.

The next step to mindful eating is to eliminate distractions, such as watching television, reading, or scrolling through your phone while eating. When you eat, *just eat*. This allows you to actually taste your food and to sense when you're full. Finally, be sure to chew thoroughly. The teeth break down food into smaller pieces, which makes the digestive system's job easier. Proper chewing also produces more saliva, which contains enzymes that further break down

food for increased nutrient absorption. Focusing on eating can increase your digestion of the food, as well as appreciation and satisfaction with the meal. This focus also helps you become attuned to your body's satiation signals.

Be Flexible

Struggles with body image and unhealthy relationships with food are not uncommon, particularly among athletes so I feel it's important to make one final note about eating for optimal health: While learning about nutrition and how it affects your body is a valuable skill that can improve overall well-being, increase longevity, and help you perform better on trail, it's important to stay flexible in your approach to food. Your identity and your worth as a person are not determined by what you eat, how you perform, or the size and shape of your body. You don't have to follow food rules or be 100 percent "perfect" (it doesn't exist) in order to use nutrition to enhance your health and performance. I would argue that the stress of monitoring every single bite and the ancillary feelings of guilt or shame that can come from eating "bad" foods (again, no such thing) do more damage to your health than eating the occasional cupcake. In fact, orthorexia nervosa is a proposed eating disorder that's characterized by an unhealthy obsession with eating healthy foods, which can result in anxiety, social isolation, and loss of ability to eat in a natural, intuitive manner. Food is made up of far more than just nutrients. It is also about connection, ritual, joy, culture, and so much more. Don't forget to bring these experiences into how you interface with food. Learn the basics of using nutrition to support optimal health, and then be flexible.

ON-TRAIL NUTRITION

How you fuel your body on trail has a direct impact on how you feel and perform. Most of us intuitively understand the link between nutrition and performance, based on either personal experience or from witnessing Olympic athletes treat their bodies like expensive sports cars in the level of attention and care they give to every aspect of physical and mental health. The reasoning is straightforward: if you want peak performance, you provide optimal inputs.

Backpackers often don't give food the same attention they give other aspects of hiking, such as gear, but how you fuel your body is just as important as (or arguably more so than) what you carry on your back. Not only does what you eat determine how you feel but on a multi-day trip, your food bag is likely the single heaviest item in your pack. If you're worried about cutting ounces from your gear weight, how about cutting *pounds* from your food bag? It's possible with proper planning. Your food choices play a role in both your pack weight and how you feel when you're carrying that pack.

Over the course of several thousand miles of backpacking, my backcountry menu has evolved along with my understanding of nutrition, lightweight backpacking, and performance. During my research for my first long hike on the AT, I couldn't find any information on how to actually eat for performance on a long backpacking trip, so I looked at what other hikers were doing. What I found were food bags full of highly processed carbohydrates such as Pop-Tarts, ramen, and Snickers. As a lover of veggies, an athlete, and a biology student, that approach wasn't going to work for me. I pieced together as healthy a diet as I could with the little knowledge I had about backpacking food. It mainly consisted of trail mix, rice and veggie sides, chips, tuna, and a lot of bars. In retrospect, it was far from ideal, and it's no surprise that I never felt great eating that way.

Five years later on the PCT, I elevated my food game slightly. I'd learned a thing or two, both about a healthy diet and how to take that onto the trail. I was vegetarian at the time, so I focused heavily on legumes (dehydrated black beans, refried beans, and hummus), nuts and nut butters, tortillas, dried fruit, seeds, olive oil, coconut oil, and dehydrated veggies. I avoided much of the processed junk and felt better than I did on the AT; however, by the end of the trail, I was deeply fatigued. My microbiome was messed up, my adrenal glands were overtaxed, and my muscles never felt fully recovered due to inadequate protein consumption.

As I was preparing for the CDT years later, my health had improved significantly and I was using an anti-inflammatory diet and lifestyle to keep my autoimmune symptoms at bay. I was no longer eating gluten or dairy and had drastically limited industrial seed oils (e.g., unstable oils like soy, corn, and safflower, which oxidize easily and contain harmful additives), grains, and even legumes (which contain a potentially inflammatory protein called lectins). I had also learned that I feel best on a higher-fat, moderate-protein, and moderate- to low-carbohydrate diet during low-to-moderate intensity efforts like hiking. This was a stark contrast to the traditional high-carbohydrate "endurance athlete diet" that I learned about in my early athletic years. With these considerations in mind, my approach to trail food got a complete makeover!

The challenge was to transfer my anti-inflammatory diet to the trail. It was imperative to maintain my health for a 2800-mile journey that would be the ultimate test of my body's resilience. If I aspired to finish the trail, I didn't have the option to eat typical hiker fare—even if I had wanted to. Although my approach to trail food on the CDT was more extreme than is necessary for most, the experience helped me to create an anti-inflammatory approach to trail nutrition (detailed next), which could benefit any hiker who wants to feel and perform better in the backcountry.

Before we explore how to eat for performance on trail, let's look at why the traditional

NOT ALL FOOD IS FOOD

What does the grandfather of long-distance hiking, Ray Jardine, have to say on the topic of back-packing food? Interestingly, in *Beyond Backpacking*, originally published in 1992, Jardine suggests that we "consider not only the whims of our taste buds but the physiological need of our bodies and brains. If our journeys degenerate into battles, in terms of lost energy and mental buoyancy, then I think those battles are usually won or lost in the grocery stores, rather than on the trails."

Jardine goes on to address how to recognize junk food in its various forms and reveals how not all "food" is food. He states that "poorly nourished hikers often find themselves low on energy and endurance. They usually assume that hiking is inherently tiring, and that the steepness and length of the trail is to blame for their weariness. Malnutrition can also manifest in the hiker's mental outlook."

Jardine points out the dangers of nutrient-poor foods and food additives: "Sugars are high in calories but they do not provide us with usable energy. Nor do they encourage recuperation from strenuous exercise, cleanse our muscles of their by-products, help repair micro-damaged muscle fibers, or help strengthen our muscles and increase their stamina. Sugars are also quite useless at promoting mental acuity."

thru-hiker diet is not ideal for optimal performance, or even for pack-weight efficiency, as many hikers assume.

Evaluating the Standard Thru-Hiker Diet

"What's in my resupply box? When is my next snack break? What will I eat in town?"

Food is a frequently discussed topic on trail. Understandably so, as hikers need to replace the 3000 or more calories they burn per day, and they need an affordable way to do so. The prevailing belief is that hikers need a lot of calories, and the source of those calories doesn't matter. This often results in hefty food bags full of heavily processed, packaged foods that are loaded with inflammatory preservatives, artificial ingredients, colorings, trans fats, and excess sugar. While the body *can* use these items as an energy source, there are significant implications to doing so.

The Cost of Fueling on Junk Food

The primary drawbacks to using junk food as a fuel source are that it's pro-inflammatory, causes extreme energy swings, and lacks the nutrients to keep your body functioning optimally and repairing adequately during a long backpacking trip. When your muscles are taxed during a long-distance hike, vitamin and mineral stores are depleted more quickly than when you're sedentary. These micronutrients are essential for athletes because they contribute to energy metabolism, amino acid (muscle) synthesis, red blood cell synthesis, and overall reduction of inflammation. The increased nutrient turnover in athletes results in increased dietary requirements. These essential micronutrients are found most abundantly in whole foods, particularly fruits and veggies.

When inflammation is high and persistent, it affects all body systems. In the short term, it results in suboptimal performance, increased muscle soreness, longer recovery times, slower wound healing, and increased susceptibility to illness. Dysregulated blood-sugar levels caused by a reliance on high-glycemic carbohydrates also affect motivation, mood, and mental acuity, making backcountry navigation and decision-making more challenging. One of the biggest impacts of suboptimal nutrition is on energy levels. Relying solely on high-glycemic carbohydrates causes a rapid spike in blood sugar and corresponding crash thirty to sixty minutes later. This leads to a drop in energy as well as cravings for more sugar. Eating low-glycemic carbohydrates, on the other hand, along with a healthy fat or protein, dulls the glucose response, providing more sustained energy.

Another reason to dial in your backcountry nutrition is that your trail food affects your hunger levels as well as your pack weight. Research indicates that people naturally consume more food on an ultra-processed diet than on a whole foods diet and that nutrient-dense food makes hunger more tolerable. The more food you're consuming, the more you have to buy and carry, which results in higher expenses and a heavier pack. A heavier pack decreases enjoyment and can lead to increased wear and tear on the body, and ultimately to injury. Of course, a hiking body needs adequate calories, and this information is not provided to encourage under-eating. Focusing on whole foods over processed can reduce the ravenous hunger that many hikers experience. As I shifted to a more whole foods trail diet over the years, it was freeing not to deal with the same level of hiker hunger as I have in the past.

An additional consideration is the long-term ramifications of consuming highly processed foods: in a research review published in 2020 in *Nutrition Journal*, high consumption of highly processed foods is "associated with an increased risk of all-cause mortality, overall cardiovascular diseases, coronary heart diseases, cerebrovascular diseases, hypertension, metabolic syndrome, overweight and obesity, depression, irritable bowel syndrome, overall cancer, postmenopausal breast cancer, gestational obesity, adolescent asthma and wheezing, and frailty." Yikes! Furthermore, Western diets (a.k.a. highly processed diets) promote inflammation via disruptions in the microbiome, the health of which is essential to your well-being, as covered in chapter 5. Processed foods also tend to be high in omega-6 fatty acids, creating an unbalanced ratio of omega-6 fatty acids to omega-3 fatty acids in the diet, which further exacerbates inflammation.

There are also post-trail ramifications for hikers who subsist on a highly processed diet for months: unhealthy habits can be hard to break once your hike ends. When hikers return home and attempt to shift their diet, it's challenging if their bodies are accustomed to highly processed foods. Cycles of binging and restriction are not uncommon and are worsened by cravings for highly palatable, ultra-processed foods. This can lead to a disturbed relationship with food and can contribute to the post-trail depression many experience.

Eating for Optimal Performance On Trail

Now that you know the potential risks of fueling on faux foods during your hike, let's look at how to evaluate and select trail food in line with the goals of optimal health, performance, and lighter pack weight. When designing my CDT menu, I mapped out the following requirements for my trail diet and used these criteria to filter my options. Whether packing resupply boxes at home or assessing food options in an unfamiliar location on trail, the following principles of healthy, ultralight trail nutrition can help you make your selections.

- **Ultralight (energy-dense):** By definition, backpackers carry everything they need on their backs. For that reason, trail food needs to be energy-dense, meaning high calories per ounce. Most hikers aim for more than 125 calories per ounce. At 9 calories per gram, fat is a good option for long-distance hiking (compare to 4 calories per gram for protein and carbohydrates). More on that in a moment. Unfortunately, this means items like fresh fruits and veggies, with their high water content and therefore lower caloric density, do not make the cut. I pack a few fresh items for satisfaction and nutrition, but fresh produce does not comprise the bulk of my trail diet.

- **Nutritious:** Here, *nutritious* refers to energy-promoting and anti-inflammatory. Trail food needs to promote steady energy by containing a balance of macronutrients that support blood-sugar balance, either within one food or when combined properly. I also seek out options that will actively combat inflammation rather than contribute to it. This means focusing on nutrient density and the same anti-inflammatory eating principles outlined earlier, adapted to the constraints of backpacking.

- **Packable:** Backpacking food must be compact and remain edible for days without refrigeration. It must withstand being squished in a food bag in the middle of a pack without causing a mess. Packaging should be minimal, light, and compact. Cans of beans, glass jars of nut butter, and condiments in thick plastic bottles do not meet this criterion. For potentially messy items such as olive oil, I find single serve packets to be ideal.

- **Appealing:** It's miserable to reach the top of a big climb feeling famished, only to open your pack to a bag full of unappetizing food. Just like with the food you eat at home, the food you eat on trail should be delicious. By carrying a variety of textures and flavors, you can ensure you'll be excited every time you open your food bag for a snack.

Heather Tip

I include fresh items in my pack to be eaten within the first day or so out of town. While this makes my food bag much heavier initially, it also extends my access to quality town food. My favorite fresh item to carry is avocado. Other items that are prone to spoilage can keep surprisingly well for up to a day when stored in the center of the backpack. These include things like tofu and soft cheeses (e.g., cream or cottage cheese). I recommend listening to your cravings for fresh, whole foods and consuming them in town and also on trail as much as possible.

- **Simple:** There are so many logistics to consider pre-hike that finding a way to make healthy, ultralight eating easy is a priority for me. You may have a different preference on how much food preparation you prefer to do ahead of time, but most of the options you'll find suggested in my sample recipes (see Additional Resources) contain only a handful of ingredients that can be found in most stores or purchased in bulk and easily assembled at home.

Healthy Ultralight Backcountry Meal Planning

Outlining a backcountry meal plan can ensure that you will be properly nourished for your trip without carrying excess weight. Each hiker has a different opinion on how much meal planning, if any, is necessary before a long hike. On many routes, you could wing it and still find enough suitable options to get by, but if your goal is optimal performance and lower pack weight, doing at least some planning is beneficial. Your energy and the overall health of your body are your greatest assets on trail, and they're highly affected by what you eat. To lay the groundwork for your healthy, ultralight backcountry meal plan, let's revisit energy intake and macronutrient ratios.

Determine Your Energy Needs and How Much Food to Pack

When creating your backcountry meal plan, the first step is to determine how much food you need to pack. It's common for backpackers to carry too much because they guess at their needs rather than taking a methodical approach. Doing basic calculations prevents you from carrying several pounds more than you need or from shortchanging yourself and going hungry, either of which can put a damper on your trip.

Traditional backpacking advice is to carry 2 pounds of food per day. Another common recommendation is to pack within a calorie range, such as 2500 to 4500 calories per day. The problem with blanket recommendations is that every body is different. A 200-pound man has vastly different caloric needs than a 120-pound woman, so recommending the same calorie range for these individuals doesn't make sense. Regarding the 2 pounds per day suggestion, it's critical to consider what foods comprise those 2 pounds. For example, 2 pounds (908 grams) of carbohydrates or protein, which weigh 4 grams each per calorie, amounts to 3632 calories (908 grams × 4 calories per gram), whereas 2 pounds of fat, which weighs 9 grams per calorie, is equal to 8172 calories. Therefore, depending on your food choices and the macronutrients that make up those foods, 2 pounds of food could be anywhere from 3632 to 8172 calories! Keep this in mind as we discuss why fat makes sense from a weight-efficiency standpoint for hikers. If you're going to carry 2 pounds of food, would you rather it provide you with 3632 calories or 8172 calories?

Rather than using a broad calorie range, use a BMR calculator to determine how many calories you need. As mentioned earlier in the chapter, the calculator provides an estimate of how many calories your body burns simply by existing. Use a claculator with the Harris-Benedict equation to adjust the calculation based on your projected activity level for the trip. With a multi-month trip, your caloric burn will go up as you increase fitness and cover more daily miles. Take these kinds of variables into account when planning your food resupplies for each leg of your journey.

Additional Energy-Use Considerations

Additional factors that affect energy requirements include intensity of the route, duration of the trip, terrain, weather, temperature, altitude, and pack weight. Hiking higher daily mileage and covering greater elevation change in a day will increase caloric needs as will taking fewer rest days. For example, you will need more calories if you plan to hike 35 miles per day than if you intend to hike 15 miles per day. Similarly, if you hike a section of trail where you average 5000 feet of elevation gain daily, you will need more calories than on sections where you average less than 2000 feet of elevation gain daily. And for hikes over rugged terrain, off trail, and in cold or wet weather, plan to carry slightly more calories than the estimate generated by the activity-adjusted BMR calculator.

Remember that these are just estimates. It's not necessary to be too meticulous. The purpose of this approach is to ensure that you'll have sufficient food for your trip while also not overpacking. If you're a few hundred calories over or under, it's not a big deal. In fact, it's recommended that you pack an extra meal or a few extra snacks in case you are delayed. That said, what's *not* necessary is packing an extra three days' worth of food. That could amount to an additional 4 to 5 pounds on your back!

Ultimately, the best way to learn how much food your particular body uses is by testing out this formula and gaining experience. If you follow this formula and it leaves you hungry, you'll know to pack a bit more next time. Similarly, if you use this approach and end your trip with way too much food left over, you'll know that you can reduce the amount on future trips if all other conditions are the same.

One final note on calories: if you are trying to lose weight, you may be tempted to cut yourself short on calories. I caution you against that approach. I have seen hikers do this, and they often end up regretting their decision. Hiking hungry is unpleasant and it detracts from the enjoyment of your trip, zaps your energy, lowers your immunity, and can impair cognitive function, leading to poor decision-making. The backcountry, where your safety and the safety of your group is at risk, is not the place to cut back drastically on calories. On long trips, it's likely that you will lose weight whether you intend to or not, simply due to the level of physical exertion.

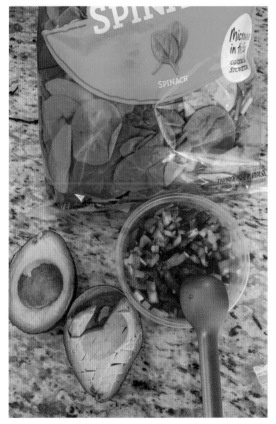

Take advantage of a town day to fill up on fresh foods.

Calculating Macronutrient Ratios for Backpacking

In the section on pre-trail nutrition, we looked at the role of macronutrients in the body as well as a method to determine the ratios that support you in feeling your best. Because the body's preferred fuel source changes depending on the types and duration of activities you engage in throughout the day, on a long-distance hike, your target ratios will change because your body is under different demands than in your day-to-day life. Although calculating macronutrient ratios for your trip does require additional planning, being intentional about your macronutrient ratios on a backpacking trip ensures you're including enough protein for proper muscle function and recovery. This process also enables you to reduce pack weight by prioritizing the most energy-dense foods and to guarantee that you're including a proper mix of macronutrients for optimal performance rather than relying too heavily on any one category (commonly carbohydrates). As with calculating your energy needs, think about target macronutrient ranges (e.g., 20 to 25 percent protein, 50 to 60 percent fat, 25 to 30 percent carbohydrates) rather than aiming for one specific number.

This section explores each macronutrient within the context of a backpacker's diet. Because you need a certain amount of protein each day to prevent muscle wasting, facilitate muscle repair, and maintain a healthy immune system, among other functions, focus on protein first. Once you have your protein needs covered, the remainder of your calories consist of either fats or carbohydrates—these are your primary sources of cellular energy. Your exact needs for carbohydrate and fat depend on you, but this section provides research and recommendations to consider when adjusting your macronutrients for backpacking.

Current research regarding sports nutrition for endurance athletes is vast, and there's an

Heather Tip
Your pack weight also plays a role in calculating your energy expenditure on trail. Since your body is carrying your weight plus the weight of the pack, you'll burn extra calories to move that added mass around. Therefore, even if you weigh 150 pounds, the extra weight from your pack means your body may expend the calories of a person who weighs 170 . . . or more. When calculating your caloric needs, take the total mass your body must move into account.

incredible amount of conflicting data to sort through. Most of the studies focus on competitive athletes like runners and cyclists, while, unsurprisingly, there's a paucity of information on long-distance hikers. The intensity and duration of exertion as well as the goals of backpackers (multi-week endurance) are different from those of competitive athletes, who may focus solely on performance for a race. Although this affects the usefulness of the data, we can extrapolate from the studies to make best guesses as to what's ideal for backpackers, taking into consideration the unique circumstances of a long-distance hike.

Nutrition science is complex and evolving. The intention of this section is to distill the research to make it applicable for the majority of backpackers. See Selected Sources for references.

The Benefits of Fueling on Fat

Energy (calorie) density is an important consideration for the (pack) weight-conscious hiker. The more energy-dense the food, the lower the pack weight. The gold standard for long-distance hikers are foods that contain greater than 125 calories per ounce, and preferably greater than 150 calories per ounce. The difference may appear insignificant, but the weight savings add up. See the Five-Day Resupply Weights at Different Calorie Densities table for some examples.

Since we know that fat is 9 calories per gram and protein and carbohydrates are each 4 calories per gram, fat is the most weight-efficient way to achieve energy density. Because fat is more calorically dense, you can carry the same amount of calories for less weight than if you were carrying predominantly carbohydrates or protein.

The macronutrient makeup of your food choices affects your pack weight, even with modest adjustments. The Five-Day Resupply Weights with Different Fat to Carbohydrate Ratios table shows how eating even just slightly more fat than carbohydrates affects

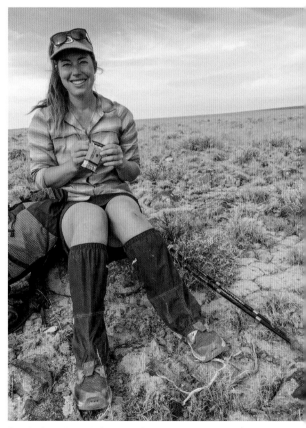

Snack time always brings a smile.

FIVE-DAY RESUPPLY WEIGHTS AT DIFFERENT CALORIE DENSITIES								
CALORIES PER DAY	÷	CALORIES PER OUNCE	=	OUNCES PER DAY	×	NUMBER OF DAYS	=	TOTAL OUNCES	TOTAL POUNDS
4000	÷	**100**	=	40	×	5	=	200	**12.5**
4000	÷	**125**	=	32	×	5	=	160	**10**
4000	÷	**150**	=	26.7	×	5	=	133.3	**8.3**

FIVE-DAY RESUPPLY WEIGHTS WITH DIFFERENT FAT TO CARBOHYDRATE RATIOS											
FAT	CARBOHYDRATE	=	CALORIES FROM FAT	CALORIES FROM CARBS	=	TOTAL GRAMS PER DAY	=	TOTAL POUNDS PER DAY	×	NUMBER OF DAYS	=	TOTAL POUNDS
60%	40%	=	2400	1600	=	266.6	=	1.47	×	5	=	**7.35**
40%	60%	=	1600	2400	=	777.7	=	1.71	×	5	=	**8.56**

the weight of a five-day food bag at 4000 calories per day. (Protein has been omitted for simplicity.) Just over 1.2 pounds difference may not seem significant on paper, but it does when you're carrying it on your back up a mountain. Keep in mind that the higher your daily calorie intake, the greater the difference in pack weight. The difference would be more drastic still if fat-to-carbohydrate ratios were adjusted further.

Based on these figures, prioritizing fat makes sense for long-distance hikers from a pack-weight perspective, but does it make sense from a nutritional standpoint? The traditional recommendation for endurance athletes is to consume a high-carbohydrate diet. This may be appropriate for competitive athletes with performance goals. But for long-distance backpackers whose goal is to complete hours of exercise at low-to-moderate intensities, that approach may not make as much sense.

As noted, the body's preferred energy source depends primarily on exercise intensity and duration. When an athlete exercises at high intensity, carbohydrates are the predominant fuel source, while at lower intensities, such as walking, fat is the predominant energy source. At higher intensities, when inadequate oxygen can reach the cells, anaerobic metabolism

takes place. At lower intensities, when oxygen is available, the body can engage in aerobic metabolism. For the most part, hiking is a low-to-moderate-intensity activity with bursts of more intense efforts, such as ascending a steep climb or crossing difficult terrain. Overall, backpackers have high aerobic needs, low anaerobic needs, and low strength needs.

Heather Tip

After exercise, your body continues to burn calories at an elevated rate. While this has been studied, there is no conclusive data on how much, for how long, and how it might vary in different groups. Some studies have indicated that this elevated post-exercise energy expenditure may last for a dozen hours or more. For long-distance backpackers, this helps to explain the "hiker hunger" phenomenon. In the later stages of a hike, thru-hikers are capable of eating astronomical amounts of calories while continuing to lose weight. This compounded metabolic increase is likely to occur no matter what type of food you eat, so you can anticipate an increase in caloric needs over the duration of a very long hike. Rest days will help lower that metabolic spike, but they will not erase it. This also has an effect on post-hike appetite and weight gain, which is addressed in chapter 9.

Consider the two adjacent charts of fat oxidation versus glucose oxidation at different exercise intensities.

These demonstrate that fat is the primary fuel source for low-intensity exercise, while carbohydrates are the main energy source for high-intensity exercise. Based on the charts, we can estimate that fat is the predominant energy source until 40 to 60 percent of VO₂ max—a measurement of the maximum rate of oxygen consumption during exercise and, by extension, of exercise intensity. Above that threshold, carbohydrates become the predominant fuel source. In other words, as exercise intensity increases, glucose utilization (and therefore, the need for carbohydrates) increases.

VO₂ max is determined by a lab test and is affected by how well trained an athlete is. You could get yourself tested to determine how much energy you draw from fat versus glucose for a given activity at different intensities. However, this level of granularity is not necessary.

We can generalize that *most* hikers operate at or below 50 percent effort *most* of the time.

In addition to fat being the body's preferred fuel source at the low-to-moderate intensity of backpacking, fat is also an optimal fuel source because the body has a much greater amount of stored fat than stored carbohydrate (glycogen). On average, most people have about 1400 to 2000 calories of stored carbohydrate in their body and 50,000 to 80,000 calories of stored fat. Tapping into the fat stores and training your body to become more efficient at fat-burning by balancing blood sugar and exercising in the aerobic zone allows you to preserve carbohydrate for more intense efforts. This is referred to as metabolic efficiency training, a concept developed by sports nutritionist Bob Seebohar.

As discussed, fat also supports blood-sugar balance and therefore steady energy levels. This results in less-extreme spikes in hunger and fewer cravings compared to diets high in processed carbohydrates. Favoring healthy fats over refined carbohydrates also supports better immune function and lower systemic inflammation.

When prioritizing fat in the diet, it's important to focus on healthy sources of fat and to avoid harmful fats, such as trans fats. Excess saturated fat can also be deleterious to the body, particularly when paired with moderate-to-high intake of starchy, sugary carbohydrate sources. You may want to experiment with smaller amounts of fat throughout the day as too much at once, especially before a hard effort, can cause digestive distress during exercise. It's also important to note that high fat in this context is recommended specifically for the ways it benefits a long-distance hiker. With any dietary changes, it's valuable to get tested to see how changes are affecting your bloodwork.

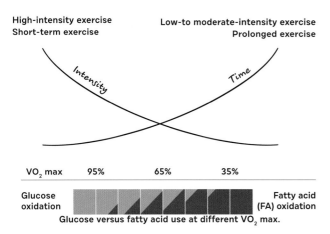

Glucose versus fatty acid use at different VO₂ max.

Low intensity exercise (up to 35 percent of VO2 max) over a long period is powered primarily from fats; as exercise intensifies, it is powered more from carbohydrates (glucose) until, at 95 percent VO2 max, glucose is the main energy source. (Illustration Source: "The Regulation of Fat Metabolism During Aerobic Exercise")

Heather Tip

There's a distinct body type that tends to develop on a long-distance hiker. It's usually referred to as the "T. rex syndrome." Because hikers use their leg muscles far more than those of their upper bodies, the body makes adaptations to build those muscles. In extreme cases, the body will begin to cannibalize what it considers expendable muscle tissue for fuel and to furnish the essential muscles with the needed amino acids. Consuming adequate protein is essential to providing those growing muscles with fuel and slowing the muscle loss that is common in the upper body. On my PCT FKT, I was barely eating any protein, focusing instead on carbohydrates. Near the end of my hike, my arms began to ache painfully due, I'm certain, to this cannibalizing of muscle tissue.

Making the Most of Your Carbohydrates

Though we've emphasized the value of healthy fats as an energy source for backpackers, we do not mean to imply that carbohydrates aren't a valuable part of your nutrition plan as well.

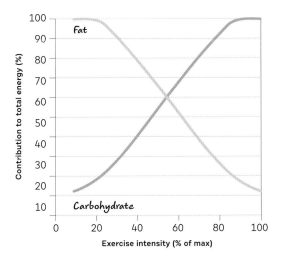

Contribution of glucose versus fatty acids at different exercise intensities

Prioritizing healthy fats does not entail eating an extremely low-carbohydrate diet or being in nutritional ketosis. As noted, carbohydrates are particularly useful for more intense efforts such as steep climbs, when muscles need quick-burning fuel. Carbohydrates also play a role in sound sleep and restoring muscle glycogen at the end of the day.

The body can digest 60 to 80 grams of carbohydrates per hour. Adding protein to carbohydrates during exercise increases endurance over carbohydrates alone, and similar endurance benefits can be found with 30 to 45 grams of carbohydrates when consumed with 15 grams of protein per hour. And protein during exercise reduces muscle breakdown. Simply put, you can delay bonking while you hike by pairing your carbohydrates with protein. Increasing protein will emphasize muscle recovery while increasing carbohydrates will emphasize performance. Since on a long-distance hike you want to prevent your muscles from breaking down and you generally exercise at lower intensities with little need for explosive efforts, you might choose higher levels of protein in that carbohydrate-to-protein ratio. A higher ratio of protein to carbohydrate will also promote blood-sugar balance.

In terms of what types of carbohydrates, you have the option of consuming complex carbohydrates or simple carbohydrates. As a refresher, complex carbohydrates are higher in fiber and slower to digest, whereas simple carbohydrates digest and are absorbed quickly. Glycemic index (GI) is a measurement of how much a food raises blood sugar two hours after consuming that food. Complex carbohydrates have lower GI values, while simple carbohydrates have higher GI values. High-GI foods raise blood sugar immediately, and then a sharp drop occurs to levels lower than before you ate. This is the infamous sugar crash. With low-GI foods, the rise and fall in blood sugar occurs more gradually.

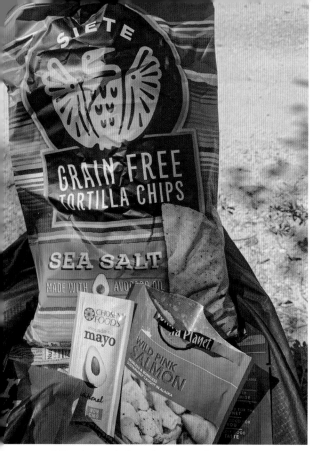

A blood-sugar-balanced meal on trail

Simple carbohydrates (high-GI) foods are great for times when you need a burst of immediate energy. Otherwise, complex carbohydrates are preferred for their ability to provide more sustained energy.

Optimizing Recovery with Proper Nutrition

Your post-exercise nutrition strategy can help you recover faster, refuel glycogen stores, build muscle, and improve future performance. This is important for backpackers, who engage in hours of activity, day after day, with little rest. in between. Your recovery meal is important, but it need not be complex, and many previous notions of recovery nutrition are no longer supported by the research. Essentially, refueling within two hours after you finish hiking for the day, and including each macronutrient, in

sufficient quantities, sets you up for a great day of hiking the following day.

Protein is important throughout the day to improve endurance, prevent muscle breakdown, and balance blood sugar; it's also a key component of recovery. It provides the amino acids that are used as building blocks for muscle resynthesis, which helps you maintain or build lean muscle. Protein needs for backpackers are relatively low compared to athletes engaging in strength sports, but it's an essential (though commonly overlooked) component of your trail diet.

It was previously believed that the body could use only 20 to 30 grams of protein per meal and that excess protein was either used as energy or stored as fat. However, this earlier research was specific to the digestion of fast-acting proteins, such as whey, without the addition of other macronutrients. More recent research indicates that faster absorption may not be ideal, because these proteins may move in and out of the bloodstream so quickly that they don't maximize muscle synthesis or maximally inhibit protein breakdown. Instead, consuming slower-acting proteins in combination with other macronutrients (such as in a whole food meal) delays absorption, thus enhancing the utilization of the amino acids. This results in a greater whole-body protein balance over time. To maximize muscle synthesis, research suggests that athletes should aim for 0.73 to 1 gram of protein per pound of body weight per day, spread over a minimum of four meals.

Ultimately, you can choose what works for you in your recovery meal each evening, as long as it includes high-quality, complete proteins and you consume them in adequate quantities: 40 to 60 grams for larger bodies and 20 to 30 grams for smaller.

Regarding nutrient timing, there is a thirty- to sixty-minute period during which rapid synthesis of muscle glycogen occurs. Glycogen

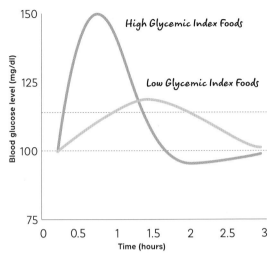

Effect on blood glucose of high GI versus low GI foods

synthesis continues for several hours after this rapid phase, though at a slower rate. Research suggests that delaying the ingestion of carbohydrates reduces muscle glycogen storage. One study indicated that eating carbohydrates combined with protein in a two-to-one ratio enhances muscle glycogen resynthesis over carbohydrates alone. Similarly, another study found that eating a three-to-one carbohydrate-to-protein meal after exercise was more effective at glycogen replenishment than a meal of equal carbohydrate or caloric value.

The popular notion that it's necessary to consume large quantities of high-glycemic, processed carbohydrates to spike insulin to restore glycogen has also been debunked: recent research indicates that the GI of a post-exercise meal does not affect endurance or performance during exercise performed the following day. Therefore, minimally processed, low-glycemic, whole food carbohydrates, along with some fruit, may be a better choice because they're better tolerated, restore glycogen equally well over a twenty-four-hour period, and may even improve next-day performance. Consuming 2.2 to 4.1

grams of carbohydrates per kilogram of body weight per hour for up to five hours after exercise appears to maximize glycogen repletion.

Finally, what about fat? Traditionally, it's been recommended that fat be avoided in your recovery meal since it slows digestion. It does slow digestion, but since it seems that absorption rate isn't as important as previously believed, consumption of fat likely doesn't pose a problem. Studies indicate that eating fat with your recovery meal does not alter muscle glycogen synthesis over a twenty-four-hour period.

In summary, aim to consume a mixed macronutrient meal or shake comprised of low-glycemic carbohydrates, along with some fruit, adequate protein, and some healthy fat within two hours after you finish hiking for the day. This shouldn't be hard for most hikers. Often, we can barely wait until we set up our shelter to begin refueling at the end of the day! A mixed macronutrient, whole food meal consumed within the appropriate time frame will restore muscle glycogen and promote muscle synthesis, preparing you to feel good again the following day. And if you skimped on nutrition earlier in the day, it's best to eat your recovery meal even sooner.

Ultimately, the most accurate method to determine your ideal macronutrient ratios is to experiment and pay attention to how your body responds in terms of energy, digestion, and recovery. Everyone thrives on different amounts of carbohydrates, fat, and protein. For some, going too low on carbohydrates can raise stress hormones and decrease thyroid function, causing low energy and slower recovery. Inadequate protein consumption can also cause muscle fatigue and slower recovery.

The foundation of this approach to trail nutrition is to consider current sports nutrition science, coupled with your body's feedback, and applied within the constraints of suitable backpacking foods. Take the information outlined here into account to determine the ideal macronutrients for you, and remember, your trail nutrition does not need to be complicated to support you in feeling and performing your best. For most hikers, consuming mixed macronutrient meals of high-quality, whole food ingredients regularly throughout the day is the way to go.

Minimally Processed Backpacking Food Options Sorted by Macronutrients

When planning your backpacking meals, consider the following whole food options sorted by macronutrients. Most foods are not made solely of one macronutrient, so they are sorted into their predominant category. You can use single foods or food combinations to meet target macronutrient ratios. Use a spreadsheet for your backcountry meal planning to make calculating calories and macronutrient percentages straightforward, allowing you to easily make swaps to hit your targets. It also serves as a grocery list.

- **Fat:** olive oil, coconut oil, avocado oil, nut and seed butters (almond butter, peanut butter, sunflower seed butter), nuts (almonds, pistachios, walnuts, hazelnuts, and macadamia nuts), seeds (pumpkin seeds, sunflower seeds, chia seeds, and flax seeds), whole-milk or coconut-milk powder, butter powder, coconut

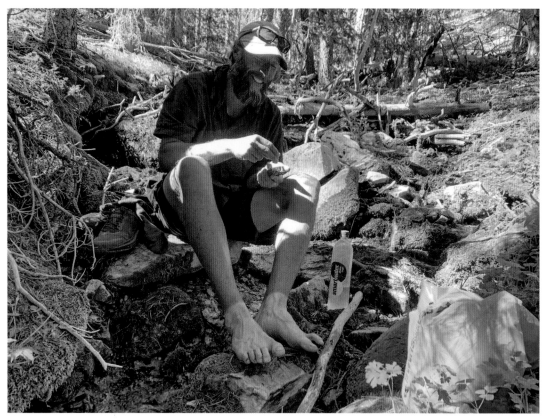

Soaking your feet and enjoying a snack is a good way to recharge during a long day.

ADDITIONAL TIPS FOR HEALTHY EATING ON TRAIL

- Include a variety of tastes (salty, sweet, sour, spicy) and textures (crunchy, chewy). Know how much variety you need to feel satisfied and be sure that's reflected in your meal plan.
- Use spices to add interesting flavors and boost nutrition. In addition to salt and pepper, consider cinnamon and ginger in breakfast dishes, and curry, cumin, chili powder, and garlic powder in dinners. Condiments like mustard and hot sauce are also great for enhancing flavor.
- Don't forget drink mixes, such as instant coffee, instant tea, hot cocoa, cider, broths, miso, and electrolyte powders.
- Pack foods that you know and like—a backpacking trip is not the time to try sometime new.
- Pack some fresh foods for the first day or two—apples, carrots, avocado, and hardy greens like spinach or arugula work well. Protect soft items inside your cook pot.
- Simplify your meals. Plan one-pot meals, where you boil water, add the ingredients, and use the pot as your eating vessel. Freezer-bag cooking is another method with easy clean up.

- Prioritize foods that are as close to their whole form as possible. Ideally organic.
- For packaged foods, the shorter the ingredient list, the better. This eliminates a lot of the inflammatory preservatives, food dyes, and fillers in many processed products.
- Make up for micronutrient deficiencies by choosing fresh vegetables and salads in town instead of (or at least in addition to) pizza and burgers.
- Liquid calories, such as instant drink mixes and trail "smoothies" (see Additional Resources), can be a great option when you don't have an appetite, such as when hiking at altitude or in the heat.
- Focus on small changes to your trail diet. It doesn't have to be an all-or-nothing approach. Some ideas:
  - Add a greens powder to your breakfast.
  - Look for healthy swaps, such as dried fruit instead of candy, and chips with three ingredients (e.g., sweet potatoes, sea salt, coconut oil) over the Doritos with forty-seven ingredients.
  - Start by swapping one meal at a time, such as overnight oats for breakfast instead of honey buns.

flakes, dark chocolate, cacao nibs, homemade trail mixes consisting of any of the above
- **Proteins:** protein powders (whey, collagen, pea, plant-based mixes), grass-fed jerky, tuna packets, salmon packets, chicken packets, freeze-dried meats (chicken or beef), nuts and seeds (mostly fat with some protein), legumes (mostly carbohydrate with some protein), non-fat milk powder, textured vegetable protein, dehydrated soy products

- **Carbohydrates:** dried fruits (mangoes, plums, dates, cranberries, raisins), fruit-based bars, granola, legumes (dehydrated refried beans, dehydrated black beans, hummus powder), certain brands and types of chips (sweet potato chips, root-veggie chips, kale chips), all dehydrated vegetables (peas, carrots, tomatoes, broccoli, corn, onion, spinach), greens powders, oats, instant quinoa, instant rice noodles

SAMPLE RESUPPLY SPREADSHEET				
	CALORIES/SERVING	FAT (G)/SERVING	CARBS (G)/SERVING	PROTEIN (G)/SERVING
CHIEF MOUNTAIN (3.5 DAYS) @ 2500 CAL/DAY = 8750				
COFFEE/TEA	0	0	0	0
TRAIL SMOOTHIE MIX	300	9	18	31
FRUIT AND NUT BAR	270	12	31	11
HEMP PROTEIN BAR	200	17	6	12
GRANOLA AND COCONUT MILK	520	21	40	11
ALMOND BUTTER	190	17	7	7
SWEET POTATO CHIPS	150	9	18	1
BEAN AND VEGGIE DINNER	500	24	17	35
DARK CHOCOLATE	250	20	13	4
ELECTROLYTES	0	0	0	0
TOTAL				
CALORIES FROM F/C/P				
PERCENT OF TOTAL				

The table above lists a three-and-a-half-day healthy, lightweight backpacking meal plan taken directly from my CDT resupply plan. Each day of this meal plan is about 60 percent fat, 20 percent protein, and 20 percent carbohydrate. It satisfied my calorie goal for that segment of the trail (2500 per day initially) and adheres to the healthy, ultralight objectives we've outlined. The total weight for this three-and-a-half-day resupply is 3.9 pounds or about 1.1 pounds of food per day. This is significantly lower than the commonly recommended 2 pounds per day. I plan for small meals throughout the day, which tend to digest better and provide more steady energy than large meals. Once my hiker hunger is in full force, I'm usually eating 200 to 300 calories every couple of hours.

This box may contain less variety than some individuals require, but I appreciate the simplicity. It makes shopping in bulk easier, and I can mix it up by rotating through different varieties or flavors for each item. For example, with a trail mix, it might be almonds, coconut flakes, dried cranberries, and ginger powder in one box, then walnut, cacao nibs, banana chips, and cinnamon in the next box.

Sample recipes can be found on my website (see Additional Resources). Note: my "recipes" are very simple. The intention is to use ingredients that are easy to find anywhere, can be assembled quickly, are suitable for stoveless preparation, meet my nutritional requirements, and allow for variety to be added by simple ingredient swaps, such as different spices, nuts, seeds, and so on.

WEIGHT/ SERVING (OZ)	CALORIES PER OZ	SERVINGS TAKEN	TOTAL CALORIES	TOTAL FAT (G)	TOTAL CARBS (G)	TOTAL PROTEIN (G)	TOTAL WEIGHT (OZ)
0	0	0	0	0	0	0	0
2.8	107	3	900	27	54	93	8.4
2.5	108	5	1350	60	155	55	12.5
2	100	4	800	68	24	48	8
3.2	163	1	520	21	40	11	3.2
1	190	14	2660	238	98	98	14
1	150	5	750	45	90	5	5
3	167	3	1500	72	51	105	9
1.43	175	1.7	425	34	22.1	6.8	2.4
0	0	0	0	0	0	0	0
			8905	**565**	**534**	**422**	**3.9 LBS**
				5085	**2136**	**1687**	
				57%	**24%**	**19%**	

Cooking Methods

Your cooking method, if you choose to cook at all, influences the food choices available to you. As mentioned in chapter 2, hikers who go stoveless pack foods that don't require cooking or that can be cold-soaked. This option can help you cut down on pack weight and is great for simplicity. If you carry a stove, one option is to purchase packaged freeze-dried meals to which you add boiled water. This approach is convenient, but freeze-dried meals are generally more expensive than other options, and some brands contain preservatives and other ingredients that can cause digestive distress. Another cooking option is to dehydrate your own meals at home. This is a great approach for creating healthy, affordable backpacking

meals if you have the time and interest to learn. A similar but less time-consuming method is to purchase dehydrated ingredients from various retailers and assemble ingredients into meals at home. This option can be tailored for hikers with or without a stove and is also more affordable than purchasing packaged freeze-dried meals.

If you decide to cook on trail, keep in mind that your food choices influence how much fuel you'll need to carry. Decide how many meals per day you want to cook and whether you want warm drinks, such as evening cocoa or morning coffee. Find instructions online for how to estimate fuel needs using your stove's boil-and burn-time specifications (see Additional Resources). Always carry slightly more than you

CALORIE-DENSE WHOLE FOOD OPTIONS	
FOOD	CALORIES PER OUNCE
Olive oil	250
Coconut oil	244
Macadamia nuts	204
Pecans	196
Dried coconut	187
Walnuts or Brazil nuts	186
Nut butters	174
70% to 85% dark chocolate	170
Homemade granola	167
Sweet potato chips	150
Trail mix	130
Dried fruit	102
Dehyrated refried beans	93

need as fuel usage can be affected by factors like wind, elevation, and temperature.

Tips for Backpacking with Dietary Restrictions
After completing the PCT as a vegetarian and the CDT on a gluten-free, dairy-free, low-grain diet, backpacking with dietary restrictions is something with which I have a lot of experience. If you follow the healthy-eating principles in this chapter, it's not nearly as challenging as you might expect. If you are on a restricted diet, or if you simply like to eat healthy, I suggest planning ahead and sending boxes. It's worth the preparation time at home to be sure you have what you need to feel your best on trail. It also saves you from having to search a new grocery store for suitable options when you walk into town tired and hungry.

For gluten-free and dairy-free hikers, many whole foods, such as nuts, seeds, dehydrated veggies, and dehydrated fruits, already fit those constraints. In addition, an abundance of newer products on the market are suitable for alternative diets and backpacking appropriate. Keep in mind, however, that just because something is vegan, gluten-free, keto, or has any other

specialty label, that doesn't make it healthy. Oreos are a classic vegan cookie! Read ingredient lists and stick to whole-food–based products.

Vegans and vegetarians should also be aware of possible nutrient and protein deficiencies. The most common vitamin deficiencies include B12, D, iron, and zinc. These all play a role in energy and immunity, and the best way to learn your status is to get tested. The other concern is ensuring you consume adequate protein; the best approach is to track your intake and plan your menu. Some vegetarian protein sources to consider include protein powders, beans, quinoa, protein bars, bean-based chips, and chia, flax, and hemp seeds.

Healthy Eating on a Budget
A common misconception is that healthy eating is expensive. Planning your resupply strategy ahead of time and thinking through how you'll approach food in trail towns is key to eating healthy without breaking the bank (refer back to chapter 2 to review resupply-strategy methods). Also, as noted earlier, a nutrient-rich diet based on whole foods often results in lower food consumption overall. This in turn leads to lower costs.

By creating a resupply strategy, you can prevent overspending in remote towns and ensure you're not overbuying. Mailing yourself boxes

Heather Tip

Many years ago, a friend was preparing to thru-hike the Himalaya Trail. She often struggled with keeping weight on during previous prolonged efforts, and she asked my advice. My secret weapons were dark chocolate and coconut, and she successfully completed the hike without going too far underweight. To this day she thanks me for the advice to include a lot of chocolate in her resupplies. ● *On my AT FKT, I ate a ton of goji berries. Not only do they have carbohydrates, but they are also high in protein percentage-wise. Talk about a win-win snack!*

allows you to purchase in bulk at places like Costco and Trader Joe's, and to search online hubs like Vitacost and Direct Eats for the best prices. Use your resupply spreadsheet to know how much of each item to purchase. Consider supplementing your boxes with snacks to eat in town to further save yourself money.

Once you're on trail, it can be hard not to spend a ton of money when you walk into a town tired and famished, after you've been dreaming about food for miles. Enjoy yourself, but remember to have a plan. If you have a resupply box, pick it up before going to the store. Pack your food bag, and use extra food as town snacks. It's likely that you'll want to eat 24/7 while in town, but lessen the blow to your wallet by snacking on food you've already paid for. Before you resupply at the grocery store, take advantage of hiker boxes in trail towns—these are boxes in specific locations frequented by hikers, such as motels and hostels, from which hikers can add or remove items for free.

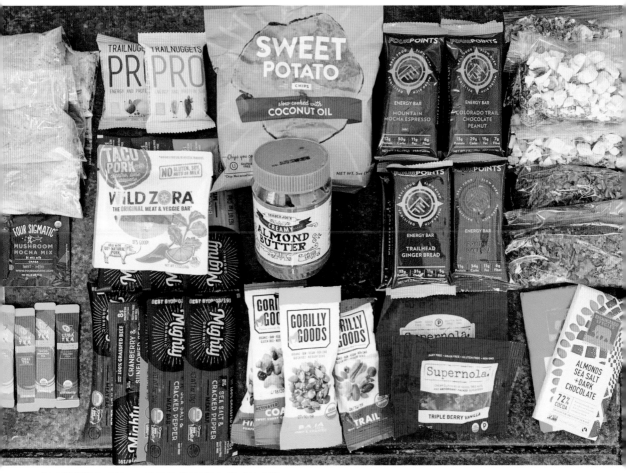

An anti-inflammatory, nutrient-dense five-day resupply

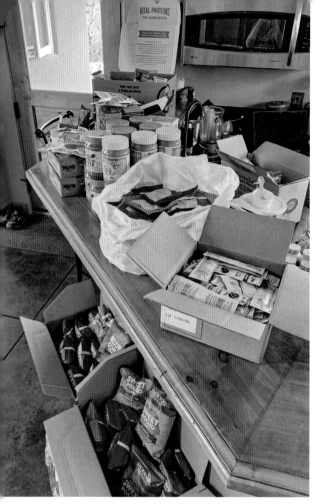
Packing resupply boxes for a thru-hike

Heather Tip

As someone who has thru-hiked with multiple food restrictions as well, I have found that the resupply is not the biggest dietary hurdle. It's town food. You spend hours, maybe a whole day thinking about gluttonizing in town. But in many of the locales, there won't be a restaurant with menu items you can have. This leads to both gastronomic and social disappointment. While everyone else is heading to the burger joint, you're desperately looking for anything to eat . . . alone. ● The mitigation strategy I've found to be the most helpful is to include indulgent treat meals in my resupply box. I send myself ready-to-eat items, and after collecting my box and eating the treat, I can join friends at the restaurant for (hopefully) some sides. ● Another strategy is to eat from grocery stores, which are more flexible than restaurants. Since weight is not an issue, you can get anything you want! Just make sure it's an easy-open can if you go that route. While a grocery-store meal doesn't make up for the lack of socializing, it does help satiate your town-food cravings and avoid giving in to temptation to eat something that doesn't work for your body.

Heather Tip

I have a less-than-stellar history with dried meals. In 2012, I did a 1000-mile PCT-PNT (Pacific Northwest Trail) section hike. For most of it I was eating my home-dehydrated meals . . . which had gone rancid. I've never been able to trust my home dehydrating since! Keep in mind that if you dehydrate your meals yourself, they may then be stored in non-temperature-controlled environments for months depending on the facility you've had them mailed to. Therefore, I now choose to purchase premade (Good To-Go is my healthy brand of choice) or to assemble my own from commercially freeze-dried ingredients instead.

Sometimes you can find gems like nut butters, healthy bars, olive oil packets, and dehydrated veggies. Be judicious, don't empty the entire box into your food bag, and be sure to pay it forward by donating to hiker boxes down the line. When shopping for trail food in town, find stores with bulk bins, which cuts down on packaging and is often where you'll find more whole foods like nuts, dehydrated beans, and dried fruit. Plus, you can purchase only what you need. Buy in-town meals and snacks from the grocery store rather than going to restaurants for every meal. You'll eat healthier and spend less. Pick up materials for a deluxe salad to make at the hotel room. Grab a bag of veggies to finish before hitting the trail again. When possible, buy from the grocery store rather than a gas station or small market. You'll find healthier options, fresher food, and lower prices.

The number-one tip for spending less in town? Limit your time there. Ultimately, spending time in town costs money—everything from lodging to food to transportation. Get in, get your chores done, rest, and get back on trail. As with all suggestions in this book, it's important to know yourself. Consider how much preparation you're willing to do, how much variety you need, and how prone you are to impulse buys. Sticking with your budget shouldn't feel like deprivation. Even small improvements in your eating and spending habits add up to big changes.

Hydration and Electrolytes

Water is essential to optimal health and performance, on trail and off. It's vital for transport of dissolved nutrients to and from cells, is a catalyst for metabolic reactions, and helps to regulate temperature, among other crucial roles. Up to 60 percent of your body is water and you can't survive many days without it. In addition to knowing where your water sources are and having

Dinner with a view on the Continental Divide Trail

appropriate treatment methods, it's important to ensure adequate water consumption. As little as 2 percent dehydration can impair mental acuity, aerobic capacity, and endurance.

Opinions vary on how to know how much water to drink. Drinking based on thirst works at rest but may not be adequate when exercising. Alternatively, drinking on a schedule can be useful, but your needs vary based on temperature, food intake, altitude, and exertion. One of the most reliable methods may be to use the color of your urine, which should be a light straw color when you're properly hydrated. It's also important to know the signs of dehydration, which include increase in heart rate, headaches, dizziness, cramping, and low blood pressure.

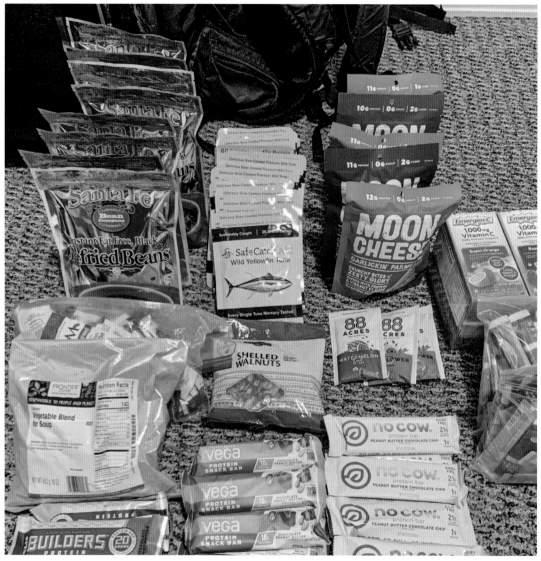

A sample of healthy snacks and meals for a thru-hike

Hikers should also be aware of hyponatremia—a condition where you have too much water in your cells relative to sodium. This causes swollen hands, confusion, restlessness, and it can be life-threatening. Prevent hyponatremia by not drinking more than a liter of water per hour without electrolytes. Electrolytes are electrically charged minerals that help balance fluid pressure and maintain blood pH. Proper nerve, heart, and muscle function depends on

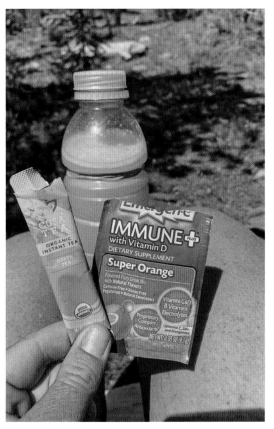

Rehydrating with electrolytes and green tea

adequate amounts of electrolytes dissolved in the body's fluids. These minerals can be lost from the body through sweat. A deficiency or imbalance of electrolytes can result in dehydration, fatigue, dizziness, nausea, cramps, and spasms. Water and food are our primary sources of electrolytes, but depending on one's diet, water source, and level of exertion, it may be necessary to supplement with exogenous electrolytes. During activity lasting longer than an hour and in extreme heat, electrolyte powders can be a great way to supplement. At minimum, an electrolyte powder should include sodium, chloride, potassium, calcium, and magnesium. Additionally, you may wish to include salty foods in your diet as sodium is the electrolyte needed in greatest quantity, and hikers lose a lot of salt through sweat, raising their needs above the recommended 2300 milligrams per day.

On a long-distance backpacking trip, it's likely that you will tire of drinking unflavored, ambient-temperature water, which varies in taste and quality depending on the source (e.g., fresh mountain-spring vs. cow-pond water). In addition to flavoring your water with electrolyte powders, consider adding drink mixes such as hot-chocolate packets, cider packets, instant coffee, instant tea, or powders like Emergen-C. When selecting your beverage-enhancer of choice be aware of how much caffeine and sugar you're consuming as well as artificial flavors, sweeteners, and preservatives that may be in drink mixes. As with your food, read labels. While some amount of caffeine can be a performance enhancer, too much can affect your cortisol levels and disrupt your sleep.

Scouting route options
on the Wind River
High Route

7

PHYSICAL PREPARATION

BY *Heather*

"You'll hike into shape."
Have you heard this reasoning before? Many people dismiss physical conditioning prior to a hike because of this belief. In a sense, yes, you will hike into shape. No amount of preparation prior (even ultramarathon running) makes you completely ready to strap on a pack and hike for eight or more hours a day. However, by doing structured, individualized workouts, you can ease your body's transition into full-time exercise and greatly decrease your chance of injury.

I finished my first Triple Crown by thru-hiking the PCT in 2005 and CDT in 2006 (having completed the AT in 2003). In the winters leading up to those hikes, I ran or cross-country skied five days a week and did some basic strength training, such as push-ups, crunches, and squats, to maintain my basic aerobic capacity and strength. I also did yoga occasionally to maintain flexibility in my tissues. My hiking partner used the hike-into-shape

139

strategy. His training plan involved a lot of beer drinking and eating in front of the computer. When we hit the trail, we were logging 20-plus miles a day from day one—and only one of us didn't have a ton of aches and pains for the first few weeks.

An important aspect of choosing a route is to select one that falls within your physical capacity. This doesn't mean underestimating yourself, but rather being realistic about your current fitness level and what level you can achieve. So if your dream is to complete a bold route, for example, make conservative choices with regard to itinerary. Embarking on a trip that is beyond your fitness capacity or developing an itinerary that is overly aggressive can set you up not only for discomfort and possible failure but also for a domino effect of incidents that can lead to injury or accident.

Start by asking yourself some basic questions about your route: Have you hiked the route before? Have you hiked in the area before? If so, what type of mileage were you able to do? It's always safer to underestimate your abilities, because if you happen to move faster, you are less likely to make rash choices than if you try to stay on pace. Refer back to chapter 3 for more on physical preparedness and safety.

To determine the suitability of your route and itinerary based on physical fitness, it's essential to understand the strengths and weaknesses of the primary body systems that can benefit from advance conditioning—the muscular, skeletal (including ligaments and joints), and cardiovascular systems. Even though the systems are the same in each person, there is no one-size-fits-all plan. Each individual has their own unique biomechanical strengths and weaknesses. Even your gait is unique to you! This section focuses on ways to build a physical preparation plan that works with your body to ensure you are ready to take on the trail.

FEATURES OF A WELL-ROUNDED TRAINING PROGRAM

Think about the ways you move: standing, sitting, walking, reaching, pushing, etc. As you go through your day, think about the components of each movement you make. For example, sitting down and standing up from a chair is the same set of essential movements as performing a standard squat. Lifting your cup of coffee is a bicep curl.

In the same way, hiking is equal to walking. However, when you break down walking even further, you discover that walking is simply a string of alternating single-leg balances and forward lunges. Therefore, at its most basic level, hiking is a balance-and-lunge act. Building a body that can do this motion over and over without misalignment or fatigue will go a long way toward preparing you for a successful hike of any duration.

Now, before you start doing lunges all over your house, take the time to ensure that you can perform them with good form (turn to the Strength Training section of this chapter). Once you can do them well, then you can begin to work up to completing them multiple times without compromising that form.

The first step toward building an individual training program is to start thinking about the components of your daily movements and noticing which components prove more difficult than others. To facilitate this process, here's an assignment: Make a list of daily movements broken down into their components. If possible, do the same for a short hike or overnight camping trip. Your list might include things like hiking uphill = forward lunges; putting away groceries = squat + lift; getting up off the couch = squat. Once you have a list, highlight the component moves that are the hardest for you to complete or the ones that are the most tiring when you do them repeatedly. The goal of your training program will be making those components easier.

Endurance, Strength, and Mobility

Preparing yourself physically for a long-distance hike requires training your body as a whole by establishing movement patterns that increase your endurance, strength, and the mobility of your joints. Many people focus on building endurance for a hike, and while this component is important, it is not necessarily the piece that will require the most focus in your program. Remember the line "You'll hike into shape"? This applies the most to endurance. With a proper aerobic base and prepared musculoskeletal system, you'll be able to increase your mileage rapidly on trail.

A common question I've encountered when training people for a long-distance hike is "How strong do I need to be? I'm just walking." Strength training is not about being able to bench-press a certain weight, it's about making sure that the muscles that will be engaged in the majority of movement on trail, as well as their supporting and counterbalancing muscles, are strong and functional enough to move you and the load you carry.

We've already discussed component exercises and how hiking is a series of balancing and lunging. What other hiking-specific component moves have you identified during your assignment? Perhaps you noticed that when you pack up in the morning and lift your pack to put it on, you engage in a dead lift and torso rotation. Or that when you're hiking, your chest muscles tighten to pull the backpack load uphill, similar to a push-up. Maybe you noticed that your low back contracts in order to keep your pelvis centered underneath your torso so that you don't topple over, in much the same way it does during a backbend like cobra asana in yoga. Climbing into the back of a pickup that's giving you a ride into town engages your oblique, abdominal, and back muscles as you throw your pack in and climb up, similar to a torso twist and toss. As you can see, the component moves are extensive!

With every movement, there are active muscles and those that function in opposition. When you're sitting, your hip flexors shorten while your glutes lengthen. Think about the compounded implications of this when you hike uphill and your glutes need to contract to push you up. If they are weak from being in a stretched and unengaged position for many hours a day, they may not be able to activate when you need them to. Strengthening the right muscles in the right ways is what is important to prepare you for a long hike.

As for mobility, it's not just whether you can touch your toes. In fact, excessive flexibility can lead to injury on trail. What's more important is that your joints are able to move through their entire range of motion. This keeps your body from compensating for immobile joints. Compensatory injuries are among the most common injuries hikers sustain.

Finding the Right Balance of Activities

Identifying what combination of endurance, strength, and mobility training you need in your plan is the key to success . . . and also completely individualized. Again, there is no one-size-fits-all plan. The movements and suggestions that follow are basics to get you started (find more suggestions online; see Additional Resources). No one movement is crucial. Take what works for you and leave the rest.

To get started, think about injuries you're prone to and find any patterns: Are they all on one side? Are you prone to pulls in certain muscles? Pain in certain joints? Frequently rolled ankles? Compare with the results of the daily movements–components assignment and look for any commonalities there as well. This biofeedback should provide insight into which body systems, areas, and movements you may need to work on in each of the primary categories: strength, mobility, and endurance.

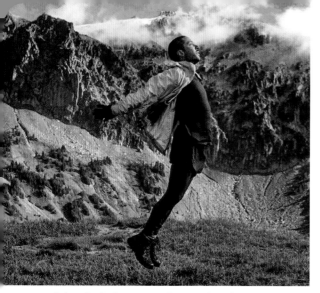

Being physically prepared for your hike will have you feeling lighter on your feet! (Photo by Tommy Corey)

Also start thinking about how much time each day you spend moving around. Long-distance hiking is full-time exercise. Chances are you're currently pretty sedentary by comparison. Look for opportunities to move more. This can be as simple as parking at the outskirts of a parking lot, taking the stairs, not using a remote control for anything, or making multiple trips to the car to bring in the groceries.

Integrating additional movement into your regular schedule helps your body to begin adapting to moving a lot more. It also can help you pinpoint areas that may need additional focus and training. For example, does standing or sitting cause pain or stiffness in your joints? Does movement ease it?

Unfortunately, most of us spend an inordinate amount of the day sitting—whether in the car, at a desk, or on the couch. But human beings are meant to move! One of the reasons thru-hiking is so attractive is that it puts our bodies to work doing what is very natural: moving at low intensity for many hours per day. Now that we spend so much of our time not moving, we've lost our innate connection and internal desire to engage in prolonged movement, and this makes pre-hike exercise even more critical. Switching

from sitting for forty-plus hours a week to walking for forty-plus hours a week is a tremendous 180-degree shift! No matter the amount of preparation you do, there will be an adjustment period when you hit the trail; proper training will make that transition smoother.

As you prepare physically—and during your first weeks on trail—remember that you are asking your body to do a lot. It's completely capable of making the adaptation, but employ patience and listen to your body as you increase the frequency in which you move. And thank it daily for what it's doing to help you achieve your dreams.

Endurance Training

Endurance training will help you make that shift to long hours of walking. If you are already an active runner, cyclist, or walker/hiker who spends ten or more hours a week engaging in moderate aerobic activity, then you may not need to focus as much on building endurance as someone who currently engages in aerobic exercise infrequently or not at all.

Aerobic exercise is simply any cardiovascular conditioning exercise. Activities that raise your respiratory rate and can be maintained for prolonged periods of time are aerobic. Exercises that leave you gasping for breath are likely approaching anaerobic exercise levels and are done at a much higher intensity than needed to increase your endurance for backpacking. Though anaerobic conditioning may benefit those who are already in strong aerobic shape, our focus is on moderate aerobic conditioning.

One of the most obvious ways to increase cardiovascular conditioning and the one that most people turn to in preparation for their hike is running. This is an excellent aerobic exercise that uses the same muscle groups and joints as hiking does. It also prepares the body for high impact and is easy to do just about anywhere without special equipment other than a proper pair of athletic shoes. I maintain my aerobic capacity in the off season by running. However, please bear in mind that running is not a one-to-one analog for hiking.

Though it might seem obvious, over and over I see runners who get injured while backpacking and vice versa. The reason is sport-specificity. While both running and hiking use the legs and lungs to move you along (and often up), they do so differently: There is more impact and faster engagement of the muscle fibers when running. There is a significant difference in the amount of balance needed when wearing a pack. The list goes on. While running is a great way to train your cardiovascular system for a long hike, don't assume that your body will be ready to put on a 20-pound (or more!) backpack and move without an adaptation period.

While any aerobic exercise, such as swimming, will train the cardiovascular system, I encourage people preparing for their hikes to choose running, walking, or hiking as their method for the endurance-training component as these will also work your strength and mobility in a very sport-specific way. This allows you to spend less time overall engaging in physical preparation. However, if time doesn't allow you to train by hiking or if you simply despise running, choose something different! Cycling, swimming, and aerobics classes, among other activities, all work for training the cardiovascular system. Just keep in mind you'll need to spend extra time in the strength and mobility sessions. Whatever activity you choose, be certain that it keeps your respiration and heart rate up for a prolonged duration and that it is something you can do for many hours a week. Feel free to mix and match types of aerobic activity as well!

Specificity training is key to preparing yourself for hiking and avoiding injury. While some people may have the luxury of spending many hours hiking with their full packs prior to departure, a good deal will not. Thus, it's critical to find alternative ways to increase your load-bearing

ability, improve your cardiovascular system, and prepare your joints and ligaments for the rapid weight gain that occurs when backpacking. "Wait . . . rapid weight gain?! I thought I was going to lose weight while on trail?" Yes, your body probably will. To your muscles and joints, however, putting on that backpack is the same as gaining that much weight—albeit poorly distributed on your frame—overnight.

Strength Training

To build a solid strength-training plan that works for your body, you'll want to refer to the component exercises list you've developed. The exercises needed to prepare your body for the rigors of hiking do not require fancy equipment or difficult moves. After all, backpacking is a very simple activity that builds on intrinsic human movements. I recommend always starting with your bodyweight alone. In the end, the ability to move our own mass around without injury is the most important strength skill. Only when you can perform every component movement flawlessly does adding weight become appropriate. Since the objective of this book is to prepare you for backpacking, I recommend you use your backpack as a weighted training tool when appropriate. This strategy is covered in the plan-building stage of this chapter.

Strength training in this context is not about building huge muscles. Instead, it's about building strong muscles while correcting imbalanced musculature. Backpacking is done on rough terrain, and your feet land in a variety of positions as you negotiate roots, rocks, and other obstacles. Your body follows your feet, so it's important to focus on strengthening every facet of muscles in your legs: laterally, medially, posteriorly, and anteriorly.

The following list of exercises are component moves—simple isolation exercises—to improve your overall muscular strength and stability for backpacking. How many of these were on your list already?

Movement 1: Leg Circles

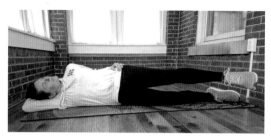

This move strengthens the outer hip complex and can help prevent iliotibial (IT) band syndrome which often manifests as pain in the outer knee (see Overuse Injuries in this chapter). In our forward-movement-driven lifestyle, the muscles of the outer hip, such as the gluteus medius, are often quite weak. Engaging in lateral movements can activate those muscles and correct imbalances. Leg circles focus on lateral hip strengthening.

1. Lie on one side with both legs slightly bent. Recline your head all the way down to the top of your extended arm, or prop it on your elbow, whichever feels more stable to you. Your top hand can rest lightly on the floor in front of your torso as a kickstand, but do not put significant weight on it.
2. Engage your core and ensure your hips are stacked one on top of the other. Straighten your upper leg and slowly rotate it in tiny circles without tilting your body forward or backward. You may be surprised at how fast you get tired!
3. Work up to doing circles for 30 seconds one way, then reverse for another 30 seconds. Repeat on the other side.

Progression: As you get stronger, increase the duration of time and experiment with size of circles.
Regression: If you're not stable enough to extend your leg, keep both knees bent. With your feet together, open your knees apart. This is the classic "clamshell" move. Progress to circles when you can do the clamshells easily without losing balance.

Movement 2: Calf Raises

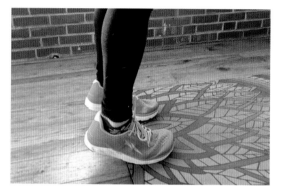

This movement strengthens the calf muscles-Calves are often overlooked, but they are major propellers for forward (and upward!) movement. They are also absorbers of the impact of each step you take. Having strong calves is crucial to pushing yourself uphill and maintaining balance while walking over rough terrain. Calf raises focus on posterior lower leg strengthening.

1. Do this move without shoes if you can. Standing with your feet hip-width apart, engage your calves to lift up onto the balls of your feet.
2. Slowly lower down and repeat 10 to 20 times.

Progressions:

1. Try one leg at a time, holding the other foot slightly off the floor. It's important with single-leg progressions that your hips remain square and balanced. If one hip sways out to the side or your pelvis wobbles forward and back, then lower the toes of the other foot back to the floor. Reduce

the amount of weight in the nonworking toes slowly until you can perform single-leg calf raises with a stable form.

2. Move to bent-knee single-calf raises. These are the same as single-leg calf raises except that the working leg should be slightly bent.

3. Move to a step. Start with double-leg calf raises and work toward single-leg calf raises. The heels of your feet will hang off the back of the step so the range of motion your calves go through is longer.

Movement 3: Locust

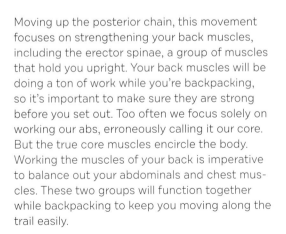

Moving up the posterior chain, this movement focuses on strengthening your back muscles, including the erector spinae, a group of muscles that hold you upright. Your back muscles will be doing a ton of work while you're backpacking, so it's important to make sure they are strong before you set out. Too often we focus solely on working our abs, erroneously calling it our core. But the true core muscles encircle the body. Working the muscles of your back is imperative to balance out your abdominals and chest muscles. These two groups will function together while backpacking to keep you moving along the trail easily.

1. Lie facedown with your arms along your sides. Throughout the exercise, keep your neck neutral and in line with your spine.

2. Engage your back muscles and lift your head, chest, arms, and legs off the floor. Make sure your legs don't splay open. Keep your toes pointed down at the mat. Hold for 10 seconds, lower, and repeat. Work toward 10 repetitions.

Progressions:

1. Clasp your hands behind the small of your back. Raise your head, chest, and arms. Add your legs when you are ready.

2. Extend your arms out in front of you. Raise your head, chest, and arms. Add your legs when you are ready.

Regression: Keep your legs on the floor and just raise your head, chest, and arms.

Katie Tip

While all components of a training plan help me get ready for a big hike, I've found training specificity to have an exceptionally large positive impact on my overall readiness. Before the AT, my training included running and biking, but I didn't do any backpacking trips. When I hit the trail, I experienced a good deal of soreness the first two weeks as my body adjusted to carrying a pack and traveling over uneven terrain. Before the PCT and CDT, however, I made a point to do a few overnight trips, hike on more diverse terrain, and train with my pack on even when I couldn't go out overnight. Including that specificity as part of my training significantly eased my transition into full-time movement once on trail.

Movement 4: Toe Raises

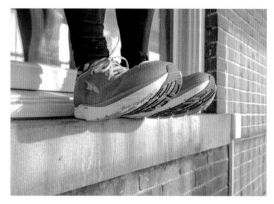

Anyone who's ever had shin splints can tell you that they are awful and potentially hike-ending. The small tibialis muscles (anterior and posterior) that run along the shin bone are often-overlooked leg muscles, until they are inflamed. By doing this basic exercise, along with weight-bearing aerobic training, you can condition them to more readily withstand the repetitive stress of backpacking. Toe raises focus on strengthening the anterior lower leg.

1. Stand on a step, with your heels on the step and your toes hanging off (you can hold a wall or railing for balance).
2. With your legs straight, point your toes downward as far as you can, then lift them up as far as you can. Repeat as many times as you can in 30 seconds. Do them rapidly, but with full extension and flexion.
3. Bend your knees at a 45-degree angle (about halfway to a seated position). Without pausing to rest, do another 30 seconds of flexing up and down in that position for a total of 1 minute of movement.

Progression: Increase the repetitions and/or duration.
Regression: Decrease the repetitions and/or duration.

Movement 5: Lying Hip Adduction

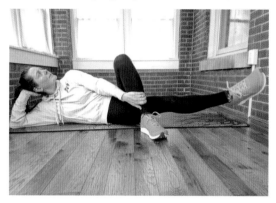

Another equally overlooked group of muscles are the adductors, or the inner thigh. This group is responsible for moving your leg inward across your body. Adductors are the opposition muscles to the outer hip (abductors) we worked in movement 1 (leg circles), and together they help maintain alignment in the hips and knees throughout lower-body movements such as hiking and running. Lying hip adduction focuses on medial strengthening.

1. Lie on the floor in the same position as for leg circles, but keep both legs straight.
2. Cross your upper leg over to the front of your body with your foot flat on the ground. Hold onto your ankle. Be careful to remain balanced on your side and not shifting backward onto your butt.
3. Engage the muscles of your inner thigh on your bottom leg and lift. The key is to raise it to the point right before you begin to roll. This may be a very small lift!
4. Slowly lower and do 10 to 20 repetitions. Complete on the other side.

Progression: Increase the number of repetitions.
Regression: Decrease the number of repetitions.

Movement 6: Forward Lunge

This classic move is surprisingly difficult to perform correctly. Since you are balanced and extended at the same time, your knee joints are vulnerable. You may wish to perform this movement in front of a mirror in order to see if your knee is caving inward (a sign that additional work is needed on the abductors; see movement 1, leg circles) or splaying outward (a sign that additional work is needed on the adductors; see movement 5, lying hip adduction). Forward lunges are a crux move to be able to perform properly and without compensatory action or any pain since they are the component move of hiking. This movement strengthens parts of the anterior and posterior leg while also relying on proper stabilization by the adductors, abductors, and abdominals.

1. Stand with your feet together. Throughout the movement, ensure that your abdominals are engaged and that your shoulders are back. Your upper body should be in a "good posture" stance without being too stiff. Avoid leaning too far forward or backward.
2. Lift one leg up slightly as though you were about to take a step. Hold briefly and check to make sure that you are not letting your other hip shift to the side as weight is distributed to it. Ideally your hips will remain level.
3. Step forward and place your foot down. This will be an exaggerated step that allows your front thigh to lower down, parallel with the floor, as the rear knee drops straight down toward the floor. It is not essential to reach parallel initially, especially if you're struggling to keep your knees or ankles from swaying in or out. Though the name of the move is forward lunge, the primary direction of movement is up and down. At

no time should your active knee be more than perpendicular to your ankle.
4. After a brief hold, engage the thigh and glute muscles to push back into standing position.
5. Repeat on the other side, completing 10 to 20 lunges per side.

Progression: Increase the number of repetitions.
Regression: Decrease the number of repetitions.

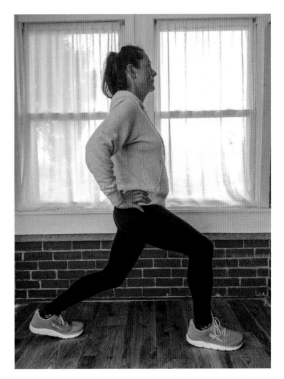

Movement 7: Squat and Lift

The final movement is a combination move. The squat and lift builds on the basic squat. Squats are the pinnacle move for lower-body strength and functional movement. Every time you get up and down off a chair or the couch you are performing a squat. Squats require activation of every muscle group in the lower body to perform correctly. If there is one move to rule them all, it's the squat. Adding the lift mimics the action needed to put on a backpack. It works all sides of the core and lower body. Initially you will do this movement with no weight. After you've mastered it, you can add a light weight in your hands or wear your minimally weighted backpack.

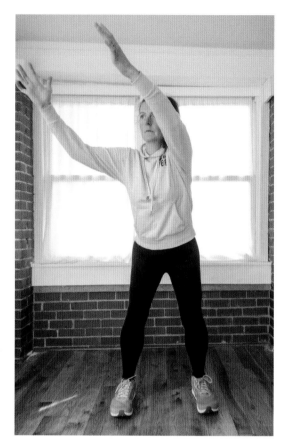

1. Stand with feet hip-width or slightly wider. Hold your arms in front of you, elbows bent and palms facing each other as though you were holding something in your hands.
2. Just as you did in the forward lunges, engage your abdominal muscles to keep your upper body aligned over your hips while you shift your weight onto your heels and lower.

    This movement should feel just like sitting back into a chair. As you lower, your hips will move backward. As with the lunge, pay attention to movement of your knees and ankles inward or outward. The thighs should remain parallel.

    Your goal is to bring your thighs parallel to the floor (or as close as you can). You never want your knees to drift forward of the ankles. The primary movement here is down and back, not onto the balls of the feet or toes.
3. Hold for a moment at the bottom of the move. As you stand, twist your torso to the right, keeping your lower body facing forward.
4. In a fluid movement reach your arms upward toward the right as though you were placing your imaginary object on a top shelf.
5. Bring the arms back to center as you untwist and lower back down. Rise up, repeating the twist and lift to the left.
6. Do 10 to 20 repetitions per side.

Progression: Hold a light weight or your backpack.
Regression: Do fewer repetitions.

Mobility Training
The third component to add to your physical preparation plan is mobility. Stretching is something almost everyone knows they should

do . . . and often don't. This is especially true among long-distance backpackers. At the end of a long day on your feet, with a roaring stomach, all the best-laid stretching plans give way to the temptation of sitting down and stuffing your face. But the mobility of your joints and flexibility of your muscles are just as important as their strength and endurance. More than that, flexible muscles are stronger muscles, capable of generating more power as they are able to move through their full range of motion.

Take stock of how well different joints and muscles move through their range of motion, especially as you engage in the component moves of hiking. A body that moves easily without impinged range is less prone to injury. The movements outlined here can be used in your preparation plan to increase your body's ability to move properly while backpacking. As with both strength and endurance, you may need more or less mobility training depending on your current physical condition. Each of these mobility moves can easily be done on trail at breaks or at the end of the day. Trail-mobility maintenance is also covered in greater detail later in the chapter.

Katie Tip

I engaged in a yoga-for-athletes program two to three times per week in the six months leading up to my CDT hike. It was specifically designed to include strengthening exercises for the abs and back in addition to other power yoga poses. When I hit the trail, my body felt much stronger than on previous hikes for which my physical preparation had focused solely on cardiovascular endurance. I didn't have any of the normal aches and pains, and I was much slower to fatigue than on previous hikes. Though I was initially skeptical of how much strengthening exercises would benefit my hike, that experience taught me the value of a well-rounded training program.

Stretch 1: Forward Fold

Engaging in a forward fold with knees bent enables your lower-back muscles to release after a long day on your feet.

1. Stand with feet hip-width or slightly wider.
2. Bend your knees generously and fold forward from the hips, not the waist. Bend your knees as much as you need in order for your stomach to touch your thighs.
3. Let your upper body dangle, clasping opposite elbows if that is comfortable for you.
4. Hold for 10 to 30 seconds.

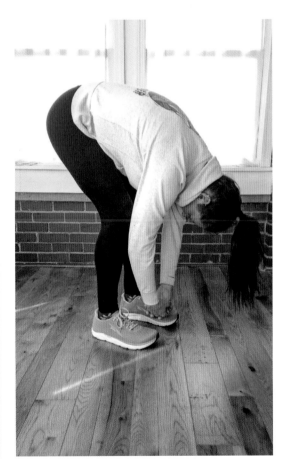

Stretch 2: Hamstring Stretch

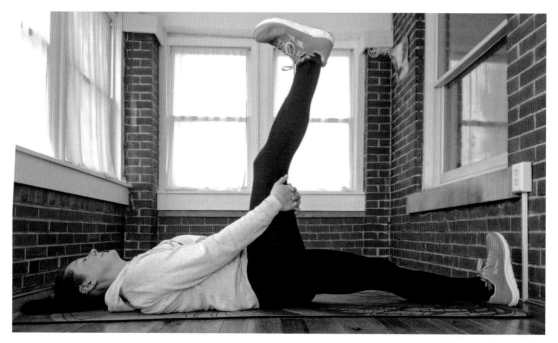

Hamstrings tend to tighten dramatically after many miles of hiking. Gentle stretching can help improve range of motion.

1. Lie on your back.
2. Keeping your shoulders and pelvis on the floor, lift one leg straight above you until you feel a light stretch along the back of your thigh.
3. Grasp your leg wherever comfortable and hold for 30 seconds, then alternate legs. If you cannot reach your leg, use a yoga strap, belt, or towel to assist with the stretch.

Katie Tip

Providing your body with good nutrition is important during both activity and rest if you want to get the most out of your training. Many clients come to me who are putting in the time to train but aren't seeing the results they want. Often this is due to not giving themselves enough time to rest and not prioritizing their nutrition. The body needs the right building blocks to synthesize and repair muscle and, ultimately, to create a strong, resilient body. This is as true on your active training days as it is on your rest days, when the body goes into full-on repair mode. Avoid restricting calories on rest days, and instead continue to eat high-quality foods in the quantity needed. See chapter 6 for more on nutrition.

Stretch 3: Piriformis Stretch

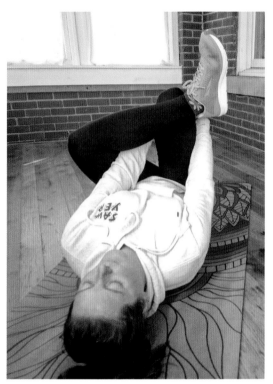

Stretching the deeply seated piriformis muscle, located in your buttocks, can help ensure your hips move well and nerves are not impinged.

1. Lie on your back, knees bent, and feet flat on the floor.
2. Lift one leg and cross the foot over the opposite bent knee. Keep the toes of the crossed leg slightly flexed throughout.
3. Clasping your hands around your lower leg (either over or under the shin, whichever is most comfortable), pull both legs toward your chest until you feel a light stretch in your rear and hip of the crossed leg.
4. Hold for 30 seconds, then alternate legs.

Stretch 4: Outer Hip Stretch

The outer hip and hip flexors tend to tighten up and cause problems when you can no longer go through your full range of motion. Stretching them can help restore range of motion.

1. Start in the same position as you did for the piriformis stretch (see steps 1 and 2 in stretch 3).
2. Instead of clasping your lower leg, rotate from the hips until your top foot and lower leg are resting on the floor.
3. Hold for 30 seconds and repeat on the other side.

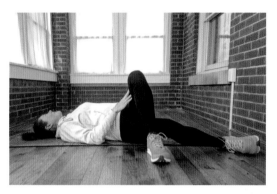

BUILDING AND MAINTAINING YOUR TRAINING PLAN

Good training programs have two components: activity and rest. Rest is an essential part of training because it allows your body the time it needs to allocate resources and make adaptations to the exercise demands of the activity phase. These adaptations are what make you stronger and faster and give you greater endurance. This section outlines how to incorporate activity and rest into a training plan that you can build on throughout your preparations for your hike. We also discuss how to maintain a healthy body during the hike.

The Importance of Rest

When I was coaching full-time, the number-one training mistake I saw was the tendency to advance too fast. This inevitably led to burnout and eventually injury. Often clients came to me because they'd injured themselves repeatedly and wanted guidance to injury-proof their bodies. Most of them were shocked to discover that it wasn't about injury-proofing themselves as much as it was about pacing their increases in mileage, intensity, or load, and resting more. The human body is an incredibly adaptable machine, but it takes time. On the other hand, living a predominantly sedentary lifestyle is unhealthy because the body is over-rested. When it comes to both activity and rest, there can be too much of a good thing!

When preparing for a long hike, it's less about being "in shape" to hike and more about having a strong, injury-free body that's *ready* to hike. If you injure yourself in preparation for your trip, you'll be starting out at a disadvantage and far more likely to reinjure yourself, compound the injury, or give up on your trip. None of these are optimal!

During training, it's important to allow muscle groups a rest period of at least twenty-four hours in between focused strength or mobility sessions. When you don't balance your activity with adequate rest, you risk developing overuse injuries. Most people benefit from a day (or two) off from all active training every week. This complete rest allows your body to engage in full-system repairs, leaving you equipped for another round of training. It's also important to cycle your overall training so that some weeks are easier than others to allow for additional in-training adaptation. On the trail, you will be exercising nearly all the time, but it will still be important to prioritize rest (see the Maintenance On Trail section of this chapter).

Overuse Injuries

Overuse injuries occur due to repetitive motion. Contrary to traumatic injuries, overuse injuries are avoidable! Doing too much volume, going too fast, or using poor form are the main contributors to overuse injuries. There are three main ways to avoid overuse injury: strengthening, stretching, and resting. By building strength, you'll be better equipped to move correctly for long periods of time. By stretching and building functional mobility, your joints and muscles will be able to move through their full range of motion, which reduces improper loading. As discussed, regular rest intervals are key to preventing injury. Each of these will be keystones in your training and in your on-trail maintenance.

Another key to avoiding overuse injury on trail is to choose proper gear. Many people think of gear only in terms of comfort or function, but numerous injuries stem from using ill-fitting or worn-out gear. See chapter 2 for tips on choosing the right gear for you.

In addition, some segments of the population are more prone to overuse injuries, including aging populations, women, and people with high or very low body-fat percentages. These groups should take extra care when conducting their training to progress at a steady and sustainable rate and take additional rest periods as necessary to facilitate adaptation.

Even if you do everything right, you may still develop an overuse injury while training or while on the trail. If this happens, the most important thing to do is rest. Pushing through this type of injury will only make it worse. If it is very painful, doesn't resolve within a few days, or you suspect a stress fracture, you must seek medical attention.

Some of the most common overuse injuries hikers experience are outlined here.

Iliotibial (IT) band syndrome: The IT band is a thick connective-tissue layer that traverses the lateral thigh from hip to knee. When your hips and knees are not moving in proper alignment, it can become irritated and tight—usually after prolonged activity. IT band syndrome often results in pain that presents on the lateral side of the knee, leading many people to assume they've injured their knee when the problem is actually in the tissue connecting the knee to the hip.

Achilles tendinitis: The Achilles tendon is the one that runs along the posterior of your leg, ankle, and heel and connects your calf muscles to your foot. Over time, if the Achilles is under too much stress—ramping up your mileage or pack weight too fast, for example—it tightens and becomes irritated and inflamed, causing pain and tightness.

Plantar fasciitis (PF): PF is an inflammatory condition resulting from small tears in the tendons and ligaments on the bottom of the foot. It often feels like an ache along the arch of the foot and results from factors such as lack of shoe support and rapid increases in weight-bearing and/or mileage and intensity. It can present as crippling pain in the mornings or after rest periods and gradually improves after exercise loosens it up. Despite this tendency, it is a compounding injury, meaning it will worsen over time if left untreated.

Shin splints: These occur when tiny tears develop in the soft tissues of your shin. Symptoms include aching and sometimes intense pain, swelling, and tenderness. Left untreated, shin splints can lead to more serious issues, including stress fractures.

Stress fractures: These are the most serious overuse injury and develop due to repetitive impacts such as running and walking. As opposed to trauma fractures, stress fractures are minute fractures that develop over time due to overuse. If left untreated, they can lead to a complete break. A classic sign that you may be developing a stress fracture is noticing an increase in pain in your feet or shins that doesn't go away with rest and seems to get worse over time.

Putting It All Together

Now that you've learned about balancing endurance, strength, mobility, and rest, it's time to build a training program that you can use to prepare your body for your upcoming adventure! Our sample training plans are made to be adjusted according to your own specific needs and goals. Customize these plans to make them work for you, and remember to adjust duration and intensity according to how you feel each week, and always listen to your body. Take time off if you feel sick, fatigued, or pain, or for unsafe weather. Limit increases to no more than once every two weeks and give yourself a rest week after three weeks of training.

To start building a hiking training program, you'll need to start with a base mileage. Since you're planning for a long-distance hike, this approach presumes you already know how many miles you can comfortably hike in eight hours. This number should reflect a distance that was fun, not exhausting, and didn't leave you sore the next day. If you don't know this number, you'll need to determine it by engaging in a full day of hiking.

Start with this baseline mileage as your weekly goal. For example, if 12 miles is your comfortable mileage for an eight-hour day of hiking, then you should try to hike or walk 12 miles a week split into smaller sessions of 2 to 6 miles with at least twenty-four hours of rest in between. One day per week, cover 12 miles in one session, preferably in combination with one of your shorter sessions. Repeat this weekly mileage for as long as it takes for it to feel easy, and increase your total weekly mileage by 5 to 10 percent from there, always maintaining the same mileage for a minimum of two weeks before any increases. Every three weeks, go back to your baseline mileage for a week in order to recover and allow your body to make adaptations and repairs.

During training, it is important to carry a weighted pack in order to condition your ligaments and joints to the demands of carrying a pack. If you established your baseline mileage with a full backpack, then you should be wearing it on all your training hikes. Otherwise, start by carrying no more than 10 pounds during training. You can increase that by 1 pound per week after the first month (until you reach the anticipated max weight of your trail pack), going back to 10 pounds every three weeks on your rest week. If you are simulating weight rather than using your actual gear, be sure to use items that will distribute weight in your pack in a similar way to actual gear. Don't use things like bricks or dumbbells, which are too dense and may damage your pack or cause you discomfort.

Sample Training Plans

Use the example training plans outlined here to construct your own using the exercises and methodology in this book. These are only samples, and the best plan is the one that works for you. Mix and match to find the appropriate approach for your body.

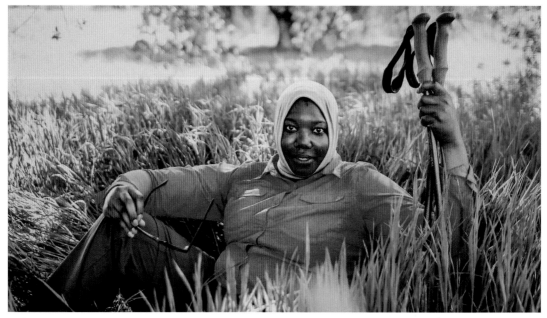

Rest is one of the most important parts of exercise. (Photo by Tommy Corey)

Bear in mind that your initial (low) baseline—12 miles in all of our examples—will be used to build incrementally toward your high baseline. High baseline is the load you can maintain without injury for many weeks in a row. Mileage increases usually amount to about 10 percent per week or less until you've reached your high baseline. Once you've attained your individual high baseline, you will cease the steady increases. Instead, you'll alternate between high baseline training, higher mileage weeks, and recovery weeks.

High baseline is not equivalent to your maximum ability. For example, my high baseline is 70 miles per week running or 200 miles per week hiking. During peak training, I may run a series of 80-, 90-, or occasionally 100-mile weeks before returning to high baseline (or lower) mileage for a rest. On an intense FKT hike, I may do 300 miles in a week, but will only be able to sustain that for a few weeks without an injury.

In general, training at a volume above your individual high baseline for more than one to three weeks greatly increases the risk of injury or chemical imbalance in the body. Everyone's high baseline will be different. The only way to determine yours is to go by feel as well as trial and error. When in doubt, rest!

Progressions for Endurance Training:
- Increase the intensity of one hiking session by adding hills or alternating fast and slow hiking.
- Increase the length of one hiking session by 1 to 2 miles.

Regressions for Endurance Training:
- Decrease the number of miles hiked at one time while increasing the number of days you hike to meet your weekly mileage goal.
- Decrease the difficulty of the trails you hike on.

Mix and match your exercises and stretches based on what area most needs work.

ENDURANCE SCHEDULE (in miles)

WEEK	MON	TUE	WED	THU	FRI	SAT	SUN
1		5		4		12	3
2	4		5		3	12	
3		5		3		12	4
4		2		2		2	
5		4		5		14	5
6	4		5			14	5
7		5		3		12	4
8		2		2		4	
9		5		5		15	5

STRENGTH AND MOBILITY SCHEDULE

WEEK	MON	TUE	WED	THU	FRI	SAT	SUN
1	M		S M				M
2		S M				S M	
3	M		M				M
4		S M				S M	
5		S M				S M	
6			S M		S M		M
7		S M		S M	M		
8	M				M		M
9		S M		S M	M		

Progressions and Regressions for Strength and Mobility Training:

In addition to the progressions and regressions for each movement, you may also increase or decrease the number of movements you include in each session or alter the number of sessions per week as long as twenty-four hours of rest is preserved between strength sessions.

Maintenance On Trail

There is a tendency once on trail to say, "I'm hiking all day, I don't need anything else." I'm guilty of it for sure! While you don't need to do push-ups and crunches at breaks (although I've hiked with people who do), focusing your maintenance activities on rest and mobility can go a long way toward maintaining overall physical function while on trail. You may find that you wish to do some easy complementary strength training during your hike, especially if you feel an imbalance forming that might lead to injury, but it's not crucial. It is important, however, to add mobility and self-massage care into your daily routine to keep your body balanced and healthy. It's also important to understand how to translate your training mileages into on-trail mileage and pace yourself in the initial weeks. Staying healthy and completing your hike are the end goals of all your preparation and hard work, so don't sabotage them by overdoing it or with improper rest and self-care on the trail!

Pacing

It's nearly impossible to create an accurate itinerary for a multi-week journey from home, especially if you haven't done a long-distance hike before. Many factors—such as bad weather, missed resupply points, or spending more time in one place or with a group of people along the way—can delay you, throwing off any schedule you created. However, having a general sense of how many miles per week you will cover and how often you'll take a zero (rest) day are important for your overall health on the trail.

Frequent, adequate rest is just as essential, if not more so, on trail as it was during training. Your body will be working hard to cover the distance and will need time to heal and make adaptations. Throughout your day, you'll have mini-rest periods to eat, get water, and deal with things like tying your shoes or layering. These add up, along with your sleep at night, to help balance out all that time moving forward, but regular zero days will be the complete stops you'll need to reset and refuel. These days will function much like your return to baseline weeks during the training period.

Many people plan an itinerary based on averages: it's easy to take the total distance and divide by the number of days you have to complete the trek. However, very few people walk the exact same distance every day. Terrain, resupply stops, weather, and many other factors lead to variation in distance covered. It's also uncommon to walk straight through without a day off. When creating an itinerary, factor in at least one zero day per week; you may find you want more than that at the beginning and near the end of the hike as well. Use averages only as guidelines.

SAMPLE MILEAGE FOR YOUR FIRST MONTH ON THE TRAIL						
MON	**TUE**	**WED**	**THU**	**FRI**	**SAT**	**SUN**
8	8	8	6	0	0	8
8	3	0	5	8	8	10
0	8	10	8	12	10	8
10	10	0	10	15	8	8

Katie Tip

Stretching and self-massage at the end of a long hiking day has become one of my favorite ways to take care of my body on trail. I was inconsistent with it in the past, but once I started practicing it regularly, it became a nonnegotiable part of my wind-down routine. It's a relaxing way to end the day, thank my body for its efforts, and prepare it for more hard work the following day. I experience a noticeable difference when I skip this before sleep. Don't neglect your self-care on trail (no matter how tired you are)!

Midway through a long-distance hike, it's common for hikers to feel invincible and push past the early-warning signs of overuse (chronic pain, swelling, tenderness, etc.). They are often shocked when full-blown overuse injuries seemingly come out of nowhere. Regular rest and listening to your body by not ignoring niggles are the best prevention strategies.

You are actually the most vulnerable to injury during the first few weeks of your hike. Although you aren't at that invincible-feeling stage yet, you're more likely to give in to peer pressure (indirect or otherwise) to hike certain distances each day, even if your body isn't ready for it. This is where having a solid training practice under your belt will come in very handy. On trail, it's important to go with the flow, listen to your body, and have fun!

When starting a long-distance hike, I recommend maintaining a daily mileage of no more than whatever your weekly mileage builds up to during your training. So if you follow the build-and-rest cycles in the sample schedule and build up to a weekly long-day mileage of 15 miles before you start, your miles per day should not exceed 15 miles for the first three weeks. Your first few days should be about half that mileage per day—about 7 to 8 miles in this example. Take two to three rest days per week (or cut your average daily mileage in half, 4 to 5 miles, on those days). This ensures your body has time to adjust to the change in demand being placed on it. You'll have time to increase your mileage later in the hike by staying healthy at the beginning. Going too hard often leads to injury, and injury often leads to heading home. After a month on trail, you will likely find a rhythm of mileage and rest days that you can sustain without injury and that feels right to you.

Stretching and Self-Care

On trail, simply stretching areas that feel tight can decrease your chances of developing an overuse injury. These movements can be intuitive, rather than structured—do what feels good, but never stretch to the point of pain. I recommend stretching at breaks as well as before bed. At the end of the day, do a longer session. While you don't need any special moves or tools, you may consider utilizing some of the mobility stretches from training if there are some that seem to work particularly well for your body.

Start with a body scan after you've eaten, when you can focus on something other than your stomach! Check in with all your muscles, starting at your neck and working to your feet. Pay attention to what feels sore or tight. Gently stretch or massage each area. This increases blood flow to the tissues and promotes recovery and healing. Even a short session at the end of the day can make a huge difference.

A company called Rawlogy produces eco-conscious, lightweight massage-therapy balls made of cork (see Additional Resources). I carry their smallest one, which weighs less than an ounce. This can be helpful for tight areas that are hard to work with manually, such as your glutes, hips, back, and feet.

Remember, your body is incredibly capable and communicative. Ask it to perform, listen to its feedback, and enjoy a safe, healthy adventure!

8

MENTAL & EMOTIONAL PREPARATION

BY *Katie & Heather*

Strength does not come from physical capacity.
It comes from an indomitable will.

—MAHATMA GANDHI

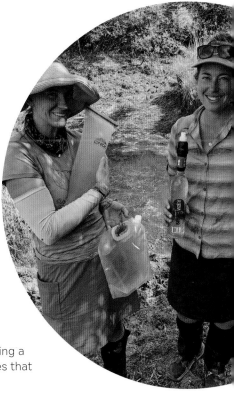

A long-distance hike—or any situation that puts you under pressure—will unearth dormant attributes and highlight both your strengths and weaknesses. Preparing your mind for a long backpacking trip before you step foot on trail goes a long way toward overcoming obstacles and achieving success with your backpacking goals. This mental preparation involves setting realistic expectations, having a rock-solid sense of purpose, and practicing specific techniques that prepare you to overcome psychological hurdles.

STRONG MIND, STRONG BODY

I (Katie) had been hiking as fast as I possibly could for over four hours in an attempt to keep my body heat up in the freezing rain. I alternated between a hunched over, eyes-toward-the-ground posture and occasionally lifting my gaze to scan either side of the trail for suitable spots to pitch my tarp. I was worried, however, that if I stopped moving even for the seven minutes that it would take to set up shelter, my core body temperature might drop to a point from which it would be difficult to recover. My rain jacket and all my layers had soaked through hours prior, and I was chilled to the bone. I was also acutely aware that my hands were cold beyond the point of being functional. I couldn't even grasp the drawcord to tighten my hood.

I could sense the panic beginning to well up in my chest. Nighttime was quickly approaching. *What if the rain doesn't let up? What if I can't warm up to at least regain function in my hands so I can set up a shelter?* I imagined myself walking through the night until I simply became too exhausted to go on and collapsed into a shivering pile on the ground. I hadn't eaten in hours because my hands were too numb to open the nutrition bar stored in my hip pocket. I tore at it with my teeth and still couldn't get to the bar. I wanted to cry. My mind fought to stay rational and focused. It was hard to remember that the day had begun with a leisurely walk around the rim of Crater Lake, snacking on trail mix while photographing Wizard Island, one of the most picturesque landmarks on the PCT.

Circumstances can shift quickly on trail. To say my morale was low in that moment is an understatement. Yet as miserable and fearful as I was, I still wasn't thinking about quitting the trail (assuming I survived the day). I had mentally prepared for the PCT to be hard. I had imagined myself walking through day after day of cold rain as I had on previous long-distance hikes. I had visualized how I would keep walking toward

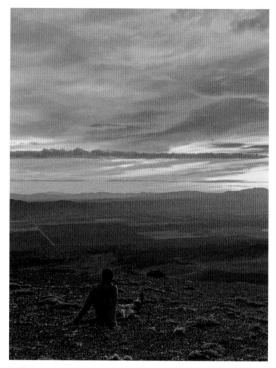

Reflecting on what you've accomplished enhances mental fortitude and helps you savor your backcountry experience.

Canada even in those moments when everything felt awful and the idea of hiking this trail seemed inane. Honestly, compared to what I had mentally prepared myself for, the PCT had been surprisingly pleasant up until that moment.

Fortunately, the rain subsided just before nightfall. I was able to dry out, warm up, and regain function of my body. Slowly the panic melted away. After a night of rest, I continued my journey northward.

We know that the mind and body are inextricably linked. This is why elite performers like Navy SEALs and Olympic athletes train their minds as much as they train their muscles. The ability to accomplish impressive feats requires strength inside and out. This is as true on a long-distance hike as it is for any challenging physical endeavor. A resilient mindset is one of the most valuable pieces of gear you can carry and it doesn't weigh an ounce.

There's nothing groundbreaking about the idea that mindset plays a key role in performance, though to what extent has been widely debated. Anyone with firsthand experience in challenging physical circumstances can attest to the power of the mind in "pushing through," and now emerging science supports what we've intuitively known. In his book *Endure: Mind, Body, and the Curiously Elastic Limits of Human Performance*, author Alex Hutchinson outlines two primary streams of thought on how the brain controls endurance: The first comes from Tim Noakes's idea of the brain as a "central governor" that limits endurance by trying to protect you, which it does by anticipating future events and effectively shutting down the body when it appears to be approaching your limit. The other is from Samuele Marcora, who says there's no subconscious protective mechanism—rather, endurance is a balance of how hard it feels versus how hard you're willing to go.

The fact that these two views are at odds illustrates how limited our understanding is of the role the brain plays in exercise performance, but what we do know is that the mind and the body are intertwined. A strong body or a strong mind alone will not be as powerful as the synergy of the two. Creating a resilient body with the strategies outlined in chapter 5 will provide you with the cellular energy for greater mental acuity and resilience. Simply put, you need a healthy body for your brain to function optimally. If you've experienced a foggy brain after a night of poor sleep, resulting in reduced motivation to complete a difficult workout, you understand this well. Similarly, a well-trained mind allows you to push the limits of your body. If you've ever done one more mile or one more rep when you thought you were at your physical limits, you also understand this.

The Psychology of Thru-Hiking Success

It's commonly estimated that 75 to 85 percent of aspiring thru-hikers on the Triple Crown trails quit before reaching their goal. That's a staggering number. So, what's the difference between those who get to the opposite terminus and those who don't? It's generally not athletic ability. People of all different demographics and athletic abilities successfully complete long-distance trails.

Backpacking is not a particularly technical sport, though it does require you to learn a particular set of skills. The primary physical component involves walking over natural surfaces with a load on your back. And though good physical fitness reduces the likelihood of injury and can make the experience more enjoyable, a backpacker always has the option to slow down or reduce mileage to ease the physical demand. The challenges unique to a multi-month backpacking trip are exposing yourself to the elements day after day and continuing to move forward when you're tired of sleeping on a thin foam pad, sick of eating dehydrated foods, and missing your family and friends. Thru-hiking success comes down to the ability to endure when things get hard. There are certainly legitimate circumstances that force hikers off trail, like illness, injury, and finances, but many quit because the going gets difficult and they don't have a strong reason for being out there. They're still physically capable, but mentally they're over it.

"Thru-hiking success is 90 percent mental." This is a common phrase among experienced hikers. I didn't fully understand it until I was thirty days into my first long hike, which entailed putting on frozen shoes and soggy clothes each morning and walking through intermittent 40-degree rain. Many of my hiking companions were struggling, but surprisingly, I didn't find it all that miserable. Not that I was loving every moment of it, but to some degree, I had expected the challenge.

My background of long-distance running provided a strong foundation for a resilient mindset many years before I discovered backpacking. During multi-hour cross-country runs in Ohio's sweltering August afternoons, I learned that I could be uncomfortable and it wouldn't kill me. Memories of those challenging twice-a-day practices were fodder I would later draw upon when my body was ready to give up and I needed to rely on my mind to persevere. Like many new backpackers, I went into my first long-distance hike believing that my gear, physical fitness, and backcountry skills were the factors that mattered most. I learned that those things are valuable, but they will not get you to the end of a multi-month journey without the mental mastery to also endure difficult circumstances. So if "thru-hiking success is 90 percent mental," how does one cultivate the proper mental preparedness?

Setting Realistic Expectations

The foundation of mental preparation for a difficult endeavor is to set realistic expectations. Having a grounded understanding of what accomplishing your goal entails is essential to preventing you from being thrown off course when things get difficult, as they inevitably will.

Consider what makes the idea of a long-distance hike enticing to you. Perhaps it's the stunning landscape vistas, being on your own schedule, and experiencing a deeper connection with yourself via immersion in nature. Whatever it is, it's likely that those are the elements that are top of mind as you prepare for your hike. And while you'll likely experience those rewards and more, it's important to keep in mind the range of experiences and emotions you're signing up for when you embark on a long-distance hike. At one end of the spectrum, you will have days where everything feels right—your body feels strong, you make new friends, and you discover your own strength as you hike through incredible landscapes. At the other end of the spectrum, you will have days where you walk through cold rain from sunrise to sunset, feet blistered, lonely, with only a packet of tuna to get you the remaining 50 miles to town.

Mentally preparing for optimal performance doesn't mean you expect to be at your peak the entire time; it means that you set yourself up to do the best you can in whatever circumstances you encounter. Mental preparation begins with the expectation that your hike won't all go smoothly. Whether you are able to endure depends on how you respond. Will you let an obstacle ruin your day (or your entire hike), or will you find your way through the situation, recover quickly, learn the lesson, and keep moving forward? Essentially, it's expected that you *will* "fall off the horse." How quickly can you get back on? This is largely influenced by your mental resilience. This section covers mental preparation techniques to enhance fortitude, but first, let's explore potential challenges you might encounter—because expecting adversity is half the battle in overcoming it.

By anticipating obstacles before your trip, you can formulate a plan so that you're better prepared to handle them if (when) you face them. Be as specific as you can based on your trip research, the expected likely conditions, and

Heather Tip

There was a moment in my 2015 AT FKT attempt where I sat in the mud and pouring rain on top of a mountain crying because I was exhausted. I will always remember that moment, because it was in this moment of deep distress that I was able to rein in the emotion and reframe it. From that point onward, I reminded myself at the low points that suffering was a mindset. I chose not to suffer. I've done many hard things and been in many tough situations since then, but I have not suffered.

your knowledge of yourself. Read trip reports and imagine yourself in similar conditions.

Physically, you can expect to feel stronger and fitter than you've ever felt before, but you can also expect to be uncomfortable—a lot. You will likely experience soreness in every part of your body at one point or another, even places you didn't know you could be sore. Perhaps you'll develop quarter-size blisters that send a jolt of pain through your foot with every step. You'll be dirty, chafed, sweaty, too hot, too cold, and uncomfortable in a variety of other ways.

Psychologically, discomfort comes in the form of loneliness, boredom, mental fatigue, lack of motivation, fear, and uncertainty. Inhabit the internal experience of not having seen another person in several days, being physically in pain, and feeling uncertain of why you started the whole journey in the first place. If you expect the challenge, it's less likely to throw you off and you begin to see it as just part of the process.

"Embrace the suck" is a common phrase in endurance sports. This approach can be useful, but what if you realize that it's not even the "suck"—it's just part of the adventure and it's what you signed up for? When you mentally embrace the challenge and train yourself to find the gift in it, you find that the very experiences that bring you to your knees are your greatest opportunities for growth, on trail and off. The difficult moments are where you get to learn what you're all about. There's no expansion when everything is going well. It's when plans go sideways and you're pushed to your edge that the greatest learning and transformation can occur. Growth happens at the edge of your comfort zone, and a multi-month backpacking trip is a gold mine of opportunities to sculpt yourself into the type of person you want to be. Ultimately, you get to choose your response in any given situation. As Viktor Frankl points out in his book *Man's Search for Meaning*, "Between stimulus and response there is a space. In that

space is our power to choose our response. In our response lies our growth and our freedom."

Your ability to reframe or shift your interpretation of an event dictates your power to respond and recover more quickly. The saying that "pain is inevitable, suffering is optional" suggests that pain is the physical sensation, which is unavoidable while living in a physical body, and suffering is the interpretation we give to the pain. From minor inconveniences to unbearable pain, you can be nearly certain that you will experience a spectrum of discomfort on a long-distance hike, including scrapes, cuts, blisters, bruises, sore muscles, and more. Pain is what happens. Suffering is our interpretation of it. We prolong pain by dwelling on it, giving meaning to it, letting it consume us. Obviously, though, if you need medical attention, seek assistance. Sometimes you have to take the thorn out of your leg and not just change how you relate to the thorn.

But don't underestimate the power of the mind and what you *can* control internally. Strengthening our ability to tolerate discomfort allows us to withstand more than we thought possible. You can choose to stop resisting the difficult circumstance and instead remind yourself that the climb will top out at some point, the rain will eventually stop, and your blisters will heal. The pain will end. You can choose to frame these challenges as lessons that build your character and strength. With this perspective and with practice, enduring discomfort becomes easier.

The Honeymoon Phase Will End

You may not know exactly which psychological stumbling blocks you'll encounter, but one you can be certain of is that the novelty that you experience in the first few weeks of your hike will wear off. During your first days or weeks on trail, you'll likely be elated over your new life. You'll have complete time freedom, you'll meet exciting new people, and you'll get copious amounts of sun, fresh air, and exercise. Each day you'll awaken excited for what lies ahead. Dopamine and endorphins will be high and life will feel good. You'll feel freer and more intoxicated with life than you've felt in ages.

It's likely that you've felt similarly infatuated with other novel life experiences: a new relationship, career, or home. It feels like the new partner, job, or location is ideal and charming in every way. You walk with a pep in your step and everything in life feels right. At least, this is the experience for a brief window of time—the honeymoon phase. However, no matter how intoxicating it is at the beginning, the novelty eventually fades. Imperceptibly, you adapt to your new experience and begin to notice the minor irritations that were there all along. A long-distance hike is not immune to the honeymoon-phase phenomenon, and it's best to expect it. It may be five days or five weeks in, but it will happen. You'll become desensitized to the beauty around you. Walking from sunrise to sunset, drinking from streams, and eating snacks all day will be just another day on trail. Eventually, the dopaminergic response wears off and you come back down from cloud nine. Be prepared for this. Simply knowing that it's coming allows you to navigate this internal shift more easily. When the novelty wears off, having a powerful *why* is what will continue to pull you forward toward your goal.

Identifying Your WHY

Your *why* is your purpose for doing what you're doing. It's the thing that gets you out of your sleeping bag and onto the trail when you wake up to the sound of rain on your tarp for the fifth day in a row. It's what keeps you taking one step after another when every muscle in your body aches, you have a quarter-size blister on your heel, and you miss your loved ones. To continue moving forward when the newness

wears off and the going gets tough, you need a meaningful reason for being out there. You need something that's more powerful than your own discomfort. As humans, our behavior is largely driven by emotions and feelings. Having a strong *why* communicates directly to the part of the brain that controls behavior. A compelling and effective reason must be deeper than surface level. It should come from the heart and evoke feelings.

There's likely a reason that you want to undertake a long-distance backpacking trip. The idea of a thru-hike probably evokes a stirring of potential within you, a deep longing for something you believe you need to experience in this lifetime. Your job is to get to the root of that and articulate it. Often, the reason involves a sense of who you are at a soul level, and of untapped potential and unlived dreams. Perhaps it taps into a vision you have for your life or a result you're hoping to attain through the experience.

Establishing your *why* before you embark on your hike is one of the most powerful mental preparation exercises. Give yourself a moment to shut off distractions, and ask yourself:

- Why am I actually doing this?
- Why does it matter?
- Why is it worth my time, money, and effort?
- What does it mean to me?
- What do I want to get out of this?

Write down your answers. Include as much detail as possible. The more emotion, feeling, mental imagery, and sensory information you can tie to your *why*, the more powerful it will be. I encourage you not to skip this exercise. It's the foundation of your adventure, and it may just be the most important piece of preparation you do for your backpacking trip. Your *why* will be a rock you can lean on and an anchor to ground you when you're thinking about giving up on your goal.

Examples might include the following:

- To unplug from the external noise for long enough to hear my inner voice
- To learn more about myself and what matters in my life
- To see how strong I am mentally, emotionally, and physically
- To become more confident; to know that I can achieve great feats
- To provide an example for my kids about the value of pursuing your dreams
- To immerse myself in and learn from nature
- To process and heal from heartbreak
- To see more of the planet before it's further impacted by climate change
- To have a grand adventure

There's no wrong answer. Only you can know what's true and powerful for you. Just be sure to think through your reason before spending time and money on a multi-week (or multi-month) hike. Articulating the deeper purpose for your hike is step one of creating a vision for your trip.

Creating a Clear Vision

To get to where you want to go, you must know where you're going. Formulating a vision of your desired destination is a powerful tool for directing your mind and keeping your attention focused on your desired outcome. With most big undertakings in my life, I (Katie) articulate what I want the outcome to look like. It's easier in some areas of life than others, and I allow the vision to evolve. For a long-distance hike, it's more straightforward. The vision encompasses not only the real-world objective for the hike (e.g., hike to Canada) but also how I want to feel at the end—mentally, physically, emotionally. Once you've created a vision for your hike, you can work on the practice of visualization (outlined in the techniques section of this chapter).

Reflect on what you wrote down for your *why* as that directly influences your vision. Your vision is a snapshot of your life on the day you achieve what you set out to accomplish. Like your reason, your vision pulls you forward, especially when your motivation wavers. I invite you to complete this exercise whether your hike is a few weeks in duration or many months.

Put away distractions and use the following prompts to create your adventure vision. As with your *why*, write it down. Once complete, keep your reason and your vision in a note on your phone or on a piece of paper so that you can reference them readily on trail. The more sensory information and feeling you can include, the more powerful it will be. Writing it in the present tense, as if it were actually that day, helps to access and evoke feelings and imagination more vividly.

Set aside your self-judgment, imagine yourself at the end of your hike, and answer these questions:

- How do I feel now that I accomplished my goal hike?
- What character traits have I developed?
- How do I feel about myself?
- How does my body feel?
- What have I accomplished?
- What have I overcome?
- What am I taking away from this experience that I can carry forward into the rest of my life?

Here's an example response: "I'm feeling so proud of myself for completing the PCT! It was one of the most incredible experiences of my life to date. I met so many interesting people and made lifelong bonds. I hiked through national forests and experienced wilderness areas that few people get to enjoy. My body and mind are as healthy as they've ever been! I experienced moments of tremendous beauty and also moments where I wanted to quit the trail and go home. I'm so glad I stuck with it. I learned that I could endure physical and mental discomfort and that I'm stronger than I ever knew. I'm more confident than ever and I know that I have what it takes to accomplish anything I go after!"

Knowing You Are Capable

Every audacious action—and tackling a long-distance hike is most certainly that—begins with knowing one simple fact: you are capable. You are capable of effecting change in your life and of doing things you've never done before. No matter what "failures" you've had in the past, what doubts you have about yourself, or what anyone has led you to believe about your capabilities, you have the ability to change, grow, and become stronger. You are capable of learning new skills, overcoming hardships, and of accomplishing great feats. Anchoring into the truth of that statement is a key component of mentally preparing yourself for the journey ahead. Starting with that premise allows you to learn and grow and become someone who can accomplish goals that formerly felt out of reach.

When preparing yourself to achieve your goals, think about the traits of a person who has *already* reached that goal. You can bring to mind someone you know who has accomplished a similar endeavor or your future successful self (the latter is the most powerful way to do this exercise). Now ask yourself: *What kind of attributes does this person have that helped them succeed? How does a successful adventurer think and act?* It's OK if you don't know exactly; just guess. You might write something like, "A thru-hiker shows up when they don't feel like it. They are so committed to their goal that they keep going even when it's hard. They possess traits like perseverance, resilience, drive, courage, adaptability, situational awareness, mental acuity, grit, anti-fragility, humor, gratitude."

Once you have a list of attributes you believe contribute to success on a long-distance backpacking trip, take inventory of where you are with each. It's quite likely that you're already strong in many of these traits. In the areas where you feel you're lacking, know that new traits can be developed and mental fortitude can be built. When you have a list of attributes that you'd like

to bolster, consider what habits you can implement daily to support that process. The goal is to identify some day-to-day actions that ensure you develop more of that characteristic. For example, if you want to develop a stronger sense of gratitude in your life, which would boost dopamine levels and your resilience to adversity on trail, you could begin each day with a list of five specific things for which you're grateful. If you want to build courage, which is the ability to do something that frightens you, make a list of things that currently intimidate you, such as public speaking or backpacking solo, and a plan for how you can face those specific fears, perhaps by engaging in the activity that scares you or at least visualizing how you would navigate the situation. Give yourself a deadline. You might even find that your fear is unfounded. Do this for each trait that you want to bolster. Each day, ask yourself what you can do to practice courage, drive, grit, etc.—whatever the traits are that you listed as the attributes of your successful self.

As you work to develop certain attributes, be aware of any limiting beliefs that arise. Often when we try to change, old stories pop up and tell us why we can't achieve what we desire. This may include memories of how you've tried and "failed" in the past (there are no failures, only lessons). It could be thoughts like, *I'm not the type of person that . . .* or *That's easy for her, but I'm dealing with . . .* Become aware of those thoughts, and question the validity of them. When you're working to develop new beliefs about yourself and what you're capable of, look for past and current evidence to support your new belief. Draw on past experiences in which you tried something outside your comfort zone, faltered, and came back stronger, or when you successfully faced a fear. You're likely already more resilient than you give yourself credit for. Revisit those memories regularly and start to identify yourself as someone who is capable of overcoming obstacles.

TECHNIQUES TO PREPARE MENTALLY

Now that we've established why having a strong mental preparation strategy is important to success on the trail, let's look at various techniques you can use to prepare your mind. Most of these tools can also be used on the trail and in the return-to-civilization stage. While not every technique will work for every person or for every situation, we recommend that you try each one in different scenarios to gain familiarity with each of the processes. This will help you to identify the mental preparation techniques that work best for you in any given situation.

Visualizations

I (Heather) decided I was going to thru-hike the AT back in 2002, when I was in my junior year of college, overweight, and sedentary. The idea was absolutely ludicrous given my physical and financial situation—not to mention my lack of experience. The previous summer I'd worked a seasonal job at the front desk of a hotel at the South Rim of the Grand Canyon. While there, I'd been introduced to hiking. When I decided to thru-hike the AT, I had logged a *lifetime* total of 75 trail miles in the Southwest and spent a total of two nights in the backcountry.

However, the one thing I had going for me that no one could anticipate—even myself—was my mental fortitude. As I began to read books about the AT, build up daily running miles from zero, and lift weights in the college weight room

Katie Tip

Sport psychology research has shown that mental practice (visualization) improves actual motor performance, although not to the same extent as physical practice. Essentially, you activate the same areas of the brain when you vividly imagine something as when you actually do the thing. This is why visualization can be so powerful for athletes!

Katie Tip

I mentally script how I'd like my day to unfold by spending at least five minutes in visualization each morning, as soon as I wake up. This is when the subconscious is more active and I haven't been distracted by the day's tasks or incoming information. Any time of day works, but my ability to focus is most potent at that time. I imagine the circumstances I'm likely to find myself in that day and how I want to show up in those situations, whether it's a challenging training hike or a difficult conversation. Like Heather, I have used visualization frequently in preparation for long-distance hikes. Reading books and trip reports and listening to podcasts about the trip I'm going on helps me create a more vivid mental picture.

surrounded by football players, I engaged in mental prep. *I visualized myself on the AT.*

I read that it rained a lot, so I visualized myself walking through rain for six months without a moment of dry. I imagined myself being cold, wet, and happy. I imagined myself climbing mountains in the mud and thriving. I visualized overcoming every hardship and finishing the trail on top of Mount Katahdin in Maine.

I rehearsed these scenes in my mind over and over. Some might call it daydreaming, and in a way, visualization is a bit of that. However, my replayed thought patterns didn't fly off into flights of fancy about befriending woodland creatures like Sleeping Beauty did. Without knowing it, I was creating solid visualizations and cementing realistic outcomes in my mind.

On the trail, I was pleased to discover that it did not rain nonstop. It was indeed difficult hiking and I was often cold. However, I never had a bad day on that hike. Because I had mentally prepared myself for something so much worse than reality, nothing ever seemed that bad. Despite all the factors against me, the strength of will I'd prepared got me to Katahdin.

Visualization is a powerful tool in athletic preparation, though I didn't know that back then.

Intrinsically, I knew that I needed to imagine hardship joined with success in order to complete such a massive task. Now, many years later, the relationship between success and visualization training in athletes is well studied, and visualization is a part of many people's training programs.

The great thing about visualization is that it is not difficult. Very simply, you imagine yourself, with as much detail as possible, achieving the outcome you wish to have in a given scenario. For long-distance hikers, this means imagining yourself on trail, smelling the clean air, feeling the ambient air and the weight of your pack, and hearing the sounds of nature. Visualize yourself happy and successfully hiking. Once you build that very concrete image, begin to swap in potential negatives: foot pain, fatigue, rain, cold, wind, etc. Maintain your visualization of a happy and successful hiker, even in these less-than-ideal conditions.

The more complete your visualization, the more you prepare your mind (and body) to respond positively to the actual occurrences. Repeat these visualizations as often as you can leading up to your hike. Include personal concerns and scenarios specific to your trip, such as fording a river successfully, having a peaceful encounter with a rattlesnake, finishing your trip healthy, etc.

This tool can come in handy on trail as well, after the initial newness of the trail wears off. Although life on trail is a radical departure from "normal" daily life, for many people, the newness of the experience is enough to keep them going. Later on in a long-distance trek, the visualization (and other mental preparation) becomes more important. As the novelty of both hardship and beauty begins to ebb, a strong set of mental skills becomes more necessary to stay the course.

Mantras

After I set the PCT FKT, a reporter asked me what my mantra was for the trip. I paused before I answered because I hadn't used a mantra, at

SAMPLE MANTRAS

Just walk.
"Embrace the brutality" (the unofficial slogan of the CDT).
Trust the journey.
One foot in front of the other.
This is what you're here for.

SAMPLE AFFIRMATIONS

I am capable.
I am strong.
I can do hard things.
Hiking is my joy.
I want to see what happens when I succeed.

least not consciously. In fact, I felt like having a mantra seemed a little silly. But slowly I realized that I had not just one mantra but several I used over and over throughout my hike. As I answered the reporter—"The record isn't going to break itself"—I realized the power that mantra and the others had had.

At its most basic level, a mantra is a short phrase you repeat in order to encourage yourself toward success. In a way, the mantra is a verbal analog to visualization. Rather than creating a thorough scenario in your head, you can summarize in a few words what you visualize.

Your mantra can be simple or more complex as long as it brings your focus to success. On that PCT record attempt, for example, my mantra was often as simple as "Just walk." These mantras came to me while I was on my journey, not beforehand, but choosing a mantra during your preparation period can be beneficial. Allow for the mantra you choose to evolve as your preparation and hike unfold.

Affirmations

Affirmations are like mantras in that they are phrases repeated to oneself to provide encouragement. Typically, an affirmation will address a specific situation or difficulty rephrased positively in the present tense. For example, if you feel like you're not fast enough to complete your thru-hike in five months, an affirmation for you to focus on could be, "My body is strong and capable of doing more than I can imagine." Using affirmations can help you reframe situations and beliefs to view them more positively. See the "Sample Affirmations" sidebar for other examples.

Meditation

Meditation is a very effective tool both before and on the trail. The positive effects of meditation are many, including improvements in stress management, an ability to be present in the moment, reduction in anxiety, and increased patience. All of these are essential in long-distance hiking!

Many hikers find sitting in one position to meditate in a traditional fashion difficult. If that is true for you, you might try walking meditation or another form of movement meditation. If you choose walking meditation, make sure that the

SAMPLE MEDITATION

This meditation is one that we use quite often and can be done during preparation as well as on the trail. You can even do it while walking!

1. Eliminate distractions as best as you can. You'll find that the more you meditate, the more distractive load you can handle, but in the beginning it's good to try to choose a quiet place without a lot going on.
2. Sit comfortably. This can be in a traditional cross-legged meditation posture, or another that is comfortable to you. You can soften your gaze or close your eyes if this helps with eliminating distraction. As I mentioned, you may be able to do this while walking, although you'll want to slow your pace and choose a section of smooth trail without obstacles. Most definitely don't close your eyes!
3. Bring your attention to your breath. Focus on the way it enters your body, what parts of your torso move with inhalation, and how it exits your body. Continue to focus on your breath for several minutes.
4. Turn your attention away from your breath to your feet. Spend a few moments noticing the sensations therein—temperature, pressure, what they are touching, etc. After a while move your attention to your lower legs. Then your upper legs, and so on, until you've reached your head.
5. If at any point you realize your mind has wandered, don't get upset. It's completely normal! Just take your attention back to your breath for a few rounds to refocus before resuming the body scan where you left off.
6. If you're doing this meditation in the backcountry, you can end by opening your eyes if they were closed and bringing your attention to something in the environment around you, such as the breeze, sunlight in the trees, a nearby plant, ants, etc. Focus your awareness on that chosen focal point for several moments as well.
7. When you're done, you can simply resume your activity.

path you walk is easy and without obstacles or distractions. Other forms of movement meditation include yoga and tai chi. See Additional Resources for some online resources about the forms and benefits of meditation.

I highly recommend finding a meditation technique that works well for you and building a solid daily practice before you start your hike. Though you may find that you're not able to maintain it exactly the same way during your hike, you'll probably find yourself in a meditative state often, and the benefits will continue.

Meditation is also the perfect venue for employing some of the other mental preparation techniques, such as mantras, affirmations, and visualization.

Journaling

While meditation and visualizations can be extremely helpful for some, they may not work for everyone. Journaling is another well-established practice for gaining inner clarity. I (Heather) find it to be an excellent method for sussing out fears, identifying mental blocks, and exploring the root of issues that may be holding me back.

I have many tiny pocket journals from my earliest hikes filled with the day-to-day of each of those adventures. Journals are great for looking back on a hike and can help you maintain mindfulness when you're on the trail. Knowing that you'll record everything is a way to keep your attention focused on what you're experiencing, rather than drifting off mentally.

Prior to my PCT FKT in 2013, I did a lot of journaling about my fears and hesitations going into the attempt. It helped me acknowledge my emotions without letting them simmer and cause anxiety. It also helped me to look at things written down and sometimes see that they were not as formidable as they seemed in my head.

Katie Tip

Journaling has been a near-daily habit of mine—on trail and off—since I was a teen. It can be incredibly useful! Journaling enhances my visualization practice by helping me gain clarity on what exactly I want as well as what might be getting in the way. Writing allows me to put distance between myself and my thoughts, which reduces anxiety or feeling overwhelmed. And I often find that many of my fears are unfounded, which gives me more confidence to take risks. Journaling can also help with goal achievement. According to one study, writing down your goals makes you 42 percent more likely to achieve them. ● I also love having past journals as a record of what I experienced, especially on trail, because it's so easy to forget the details. Reading even a short entry transports me back to that day, and I'm usually left with immense gratitude for everything I got to experience. In day-to-day life, if I'm going through a problem or difficult time, I can look back at journals to see how I navigated something similar in the past. As with visualization, mornings are the best time of day for me to journal. Find what works for you!

As mentioned earlier in this chapter, knowing your *why* is essential to success in a long-distance hike. This is the best prompt to start from when you begin journaling. Once you've written out your *why* move on to your *why nots*. Spend time journaling about what you'll be giving up or missing out on by taking this trip. Reflect on your answers and write down what comes to mind about your willingness and motivations to meet your *why* and be OK with your *why nots*.

Other journaling prompts can be useful:
- What scares me about this trip?
- What am I most worried about losing by doing this? Gaining?
- What will I do if I cannot complete the trip?

MENTAL PREPARATION TECHNIQUES AND SAMPLE APPLICATIONS

	PRE-TRAIL	ON-TRAIL	POST-TRAIL
VISUALIZATIONS	◉	◉	◉
MANTRAS	◉	◉	◉
AFFIRMATIONS	◉	◉	◉
MEDITATION	◉	◉	◉
JOURNALING	◉	◉	◉
VOLUNTARY HARDSHIP	◉		

Journaling is a wonderful habit to establish prior to setting out and, like meditation, is well worth continuing on trail. Thorough journaling about the ups, downs, minutiae, and excitement of each day can enhance your awareness in the moment and creates a touchstone to deal with post-hike depression (see chapter 9 for more on reintegration strategies).

Practice Voluntary Hardship

One of the most practical ways to prepare yourself mentally for the rigors of hiking long distances is to do difficult things. Doing hard things trains your brain to endure. At our most primitive level, our brains want to preserve our bodies. When the going gets tough, our brains tell us to quit in order to save our energy for real life-threatening scenarios. But mental toughness is key to success on the trail, and you most definitely have the capacity to do this difficult thing.

Forays into voluntary hardship do not have to be over-the-top 20-mile hikes without food. They can be simple things such as turning off the AC when it's hot and gaining familiarity with that discomfort. It can be giving up a habit such as caffeine or alcohol for several weeks and discovering you have the willpower to say no. Any situation in which you normally want to decrease discomfort and increase ease provides an opportunity to build your mental strength through practicing voluntary hardship.

> **Katie Tip**
>
> *Strengthening your resolve to do hard things is one of the most powerful methods of mental preparation not only for the trail but for every area of life. When you make it a habit to lean in to challenges, you learn that you are capable of more than you previously believed. You begin to identify as someone who is good at enduring difficulty. Challenges—on trail or at home—become easier to navigate because you've practiced them, and that practice gives you confidence. My first memory of intentionally leaning in to discomfort was going on training runs in the rain and snow during junior high cross-country. I learned that the mental strength I gained far outweighed the short-term physical discomfort. Those runs made me feel tough, which emboldened me to take on more difficult challenges. As with any of the techniques in this chapter, the most benefit will be gained from practicing them on a regular basis. Daily cold showers or ice baths are one way to practice voluntary hardship daily. Start small and build up.*

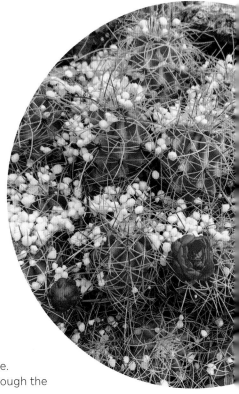

Late spring graupel falling upon cactus blooms in the Great Basin

9

REINTEGRATION

BY *Katie & Heather*

The bliss of hiking for weeks or months will inevitably end. Whether at the completion of the trail or due to other constraints, you will stop walking and you will go home. It is said that long-distance hiking is a great metaphor for life, with all its ups and downs. But I (Heather) have always felt that it most poignantly mirrors life in this aspect: it ends. And just as we spend very little time considering the inevitability of our own death, long-distance hikers are often underprepared for their journey to end and the myriad repercussions that follow. This chapter is devoted to that wild unknown that accompanies the end of the journey.

COMMON MENTAL CHALLENGES OF REINTEGRATION

While no one can know exactly which mental challenges will most affect them after a long hike, knowing the categories in which most people tend to struggle can help in two significant ways—to recognize that you are not alone and to prepare. Just as mental preparation can give you the tools to work through the

Katie Tip

In addition to approaching this transition period with gratitude, I also find patience and surrender are invaluable. After my first couple of thru-hikes, I was impatient with myself for feeling depressed and not being able to jump right back into "normal" life. I tried to avoid the difficult emotions by distracting myself from them with activities like work or running rather than accept what I was feeling. This only made the depressed period last longer and robbed me of the opportunity to work with the emotions and use them to learn about myself and grow. I've since learned to allow whatever comes up and be with it rather than push it away. For me, post-trail depression shows up most strongly as an overwhelming sense of meaninglessness. When I allow myself to be with that emotion for as long as needed, and treat myself with compassion in the process, it naturally dissipates. Further, by facing it head-on, I can transmute challenging feelings into something meaningful, like a piece of writing. There are techniques discussed in this chapter that can help ease the post-trail transition, but they're no substitute for providing yourself with adequate time and space to process your emotions.

challenges of a long hike, it can also help you work through the mental challenges that follow one. On trail, the same techniques you use pre-trip—visualization, affirmations, mantras, and meditation—will help prepare you for a seamless transition to life after the trail. And once you're home, journaling can be another powerful tool to process the emotions. In addition to these strategies, this chapter also includes others that will benefit both physical and mental health.

My first book, *Thirst: 2600 Miles to Home*, was formed largely from the post-hike journaling that I did to work my way through post-trail depression. The hike I did on the PCT in 2013 was the most difficult, incredible, and mind-boggling thing I had ever done. There were days I could barely believe I'd even accomplished what I had. Yet I had intensely visceral memories of every

step of the way. Chances are that when you return home, you, too, will find yourself awash with a mix of emotions. As with writing down your fears beforehand for relief of anxiety as well as self-analysis, journaling about the complexities of your post-hike feelings can also help you work through them.

Post-Trail Depression

The majority of hikers will go through some sort of post-trail depression period. Length and severity vary widely. Some hikers may be in a vague funk or feel out of sorts for a few days or weeks in a way that has little impact on other parts of their lives. Others may experience full clinical depression for a prolonged period, making it very difficult to function in day-to-day activities.

There are many reasons this depressive state happens. In large part, it's a product of brain chemistry and hormone rebalancing after many months of exercising daily and living in sync with natural sunlight. Some people will naturally rebalance more rapidly and easily than others. Some may need medical assistance with the transition. The key is to understand that there is nothing wrong with you for experiencing this period of depression. Your body and mind together are an incredibly adaptable organism; but, as we discussed in the preparation chapters, the adaptation is not instant. Just as it took time for you to adapt to the rigors of the trail, it will take time to readapt to a less physically demanding lifestyle. This includes all of your body systems, from digestion to your brain.

The other major cause of this depressive state is grief. This aspect is not easily understood by those who have not experienced a long hike since we typically associate grief with the loss of a loved one, but grief can apply to the close of any meaningful chapter in life. In addition, I strongly believe that the person you experience being on trail will be far different from the person you are used to being. Hence, you may very well experience the grief of losing that self once home.

Since this aspect of the post-hike mental challenge can look very different for each individual, there is no one solution that works for everyone. However, as someone who has a lot of practice with coping after having completed more than a dozen thru-hikes, I can say that it does get easier to manage the more often you do it. Going through this process has helped me become a more adaptable and compassionate person in other aspects of my life with regard to mental health and grief processing.

Approaching this transition period with a mindset of gratitude can greatly help you during the process. One effective reframing technique I suggest is being grateful for having had the opportunity to experience something that you loved so much that you experienced grief when it ended. Similarly, I recommend thanking your body and your mind for their ability to adapt to major changes.

Journaling about your emotions as well as what you miss about the trail and your on-trail self can help you identify ways to bring those aspects into your life off trail. For example, I only felt truly free to be myself when I was on trail. There I felt beautiful, strong, and connected. At home I felt misunderstood, trapped, and judged. After many years of pendulating between the freedom and wholeness of the trail and the grief afterward as I struggled through that trapped state, I finally unlocked the secret to my own happiness through journaling (as mentioned earlier). This revelation started a long journey of working through my personal baggage—a lack of self-esteem and self-love that I had previously only been able to leave behind at the trailhead. In the end I emerged as a well-adapted human who can now process grief more easily, and I've also been able to write two memoirs from my experiences on trail and my mental journey to this new place.

Embracing the shadow period after a hike can provide great insight and opportunity for personal growth, just as spending months hiking through nature can. Keeping an open heart and mindset for growth through both periods is ideal for overall health and adaptability.

Reverse Culture Shock

If you have traveled internationally you have likely experienced culture shock—the initial adaptation to a new culture. Reverse culture shock is a term typically used to describe the experience of expatriates returning home after spending many years abroad in a culture dramatically different from their own. Upon returning to their homeland, they may find it as foreign as the other culture once seemed.

Something very similar often happens to long-distance hikers when they return home. The natural world is a vastly different place than our temperature-controlled home environments and our constantly entertained, on-demand society. The early weeks on trail will likely be difficult as you get used to sleeping on the ground, being unable to achieve a comfortable temperature, and coping with the lack of on-demand clean water. However, as you spend more time immersed in this environment, you will likely begin to feel at home.

Returning to a world where you travel in vehicles, sleep in a bed, and dial your comfort easily can be shocking. For several weeks after my first thru-hike, I found beds uncomfortable. My parents would often find me sleeping on our back deck or in the yard in the mornings. After months of sleeping on the wooden shelter floors on the AT, I simply could not get comfortable on a squishy mattress! My mom also laughingly remembers the day she finally stopped me in my tracks on my thirteenth or fourteenth aimless lap pacing through the house.

"What are you doing?"

SAMPLE APPLICATION OF MENTAL REINTEGRATION TECHNIQUES

	POST-TRAIL DEPRESSION	REVERSE CULTURE SHOCK	
VISUALIZATIONS	Start by visualizing yourself at your happiest moment on trail. Make the scene concrete in your mind: How did it look, smell, taste, sound, feel? Bring together as many details as you can of that moment. Notice how you feel in that moment and how that alters your emotions and physiology in the present. One by one, replace the aspects of the trail scene with a scene from your off-trail life while focusing on maintaining the feeling you cultivated in your visualization.	Start by visualizing yourself in the most recent situation where you felt uncomfortable or upset by the off-trail world you came back to. Be as detailed as you can. Notice the emotional and physiological impacts you feel. Now visualize yourself as content and relaxed in that same situation without changing anything in the scene.	
MANTRAS	Repeat mantras such as "This will get better." "There is no timeline for grief." "It's OK to feel these emotions."	Repeat mantras such as "Things do not work the same way here and that is all right." "Change is a precursor to growth." "It's OK to feel unsettled."	
AFFIRMATIONS	Repeat reframed or positive affirmations such as "I am grateful I experienced something I loved so much." "I am synthesizing a wonderful experience into something new and beautiful."	Repeat reframed or positive affirmations such as "I am grateful to have new experiences to bring into my life." "I can change only myself."	
MEDITATION	Choose a comfortable position and focus on your breath. Imagine that each inhalation is bringing lightness into your body. Imagine that each exhalation is releasing heaviness. Continue in this way, coming back to focus on the breath when your mind wanders.	Choose a comfortable position and focus on your breath. Slowly canvass your entire body, one part at a time, noticing how each feels. Come back to the breath. Notice that this same body and this same act of breathing is continuous prior to, during, and now after the trail.	
JOURNALING	Journal for as long as you wish about this prompt: "Today I miss the trail because _____ and it makes me feel _____ ."	Journal for as long as you wish about this prompt: "I don't understand how _____ did not bother me before my hike. Now that I am aware of it, I want to _____ ."	

After a moment's thought, I replied, "I guess I just haven't walked enough today."

My body was used to 20 or more miles of walking and it simply couldn't sit still! So I went outside and walked for a few hours down the country roads until I finally felt like I'd done "enough." I made jogging part of my daily routine after that, channeling that restlessness

ALIENATION	POST-TRAIL HEALTH RAMIFICATIONS
Start by visualizing yourself in the most recent situation where you felt uncomfortable or upset by family or friends. Be as detailed as you can. Notice the emotional and physiological impacts you feel. Now visualize yourself telling that person how disconnected you feel. Be as detailed as you can. Is it word choices they make? Lack of interest in what you've done? Expectations that you or they have placed on you? Visualize clear communication.	Start by visualizing yourself during a time in your life when you felt strong and resilient in mind and body. Be as detailed as possible. How is your energy, your mental clarity, your mood? Notice the feelings and emotions, the felt sense of vibrant health. Notice the sense of acceptance and gratitude you have for yourself and all that your body allows you to do. From that state, ask yourself: How do I want to treat my body? How do I want to talk to myself? What can I do today to take care of my health?
Repeat mantras such as "Not everyone will understand me and that is OK." "Communication is the key to healthy relationships." "I am not alone."	Repeat mantras such as "I am strong, healthy, and resilient." "My health is my greatest asset and I treat my body with respect."
Repeat reframed or positive affirmations such as "I have a wonderful family and supportive friends." "I am connected to myself and others."	Repeat reframed or positive affirmations such as "I love my body and my body loves me." "I take care of my body and my body takes care of me."
Choose a comfortable position and focus on your breath. After a while, shift your attention to the most recent interaction that left you feeling alienated from family or friends. Note with impartiality any physiological or emotional changes that happen, naming them silently if you'd like to. After you've sorted through those and identified them, focus on your breath again. Label the in-breaths as confident, calm, and/or content. Label the out-breaths as those other feelings and emotions. As you breathe confidence, calm, and contentment into your body, picture yourself as growing taller than the other person or people or perhaps floating upward above them in that interaction. What do you notice about the other person or your interactions with them now that you didn't notice before? Return focus to your breath and then allow yourself to reenter the interaction, rather than being above it. What has shifted in you?	Choose a comfortable position, sitting or lying down. Take three deep breaths, inhaling through your nose and exhaling through your mouth. Feel the sensations where your body connects with the surface beneath you. Begin to scan your body from the top of your head all the way down to your toes. Start by placing your attention on your head and really sensing that area of your body. Next move your attention down to your neck, then to your chest, your upper arms, your lower arms, your hands, your stomach, your pelvis, your thighs, your calves, and down to the bottoms of your feet. With each body part, feel it from the inside and name any sensations you feel there, such as tension or tingling. At the end, take a deep breath and feel your entire body all at once, sitting or lying there, breathing. Feel gratitude for your body. When you're ready, open your eyes.
Journal for as long as you wish about this prompt: "Before my hike _____ was important in my life. Now I feel as though they are _____ ."	Journal for as long as you wish about this prompt: "Today I'm grateful for my body because _____. I take care of my body by _____ ."

into action that was good for my mind and my health.

Another common shock of reentry is the amount of stuff surrounding us in our off-trail lives. After traveling and thriving with only the possessions we carried on our backs for months on end, many hikers, myself included, are sickened upon returning by the sheer volume of things we left in storage. A complete purge of possessions is common, so don't be too surprised if you find yourself crying about how much you miss the trail as you fill boxes to send to Goodwill shortly after you return home!

Additionally, the trail is a quiet place. At the outset, I find that my mind initially races with all kinds of thoughts and worries, meanwhile feeling anxious because there is no noise on trail. Many hikers listen to audiobooks or music to ease this stressful transition period. Eventually, though, your mind begins to slow down to match your less-than-5-miles-per-hour pace, and your ears begin to notice the sounds of birds and squirrels, the whisper of wind, and the rhythmic thudding of your own feet and heart. These sounds are soft and blend with the neutral palette of the wild. Stepping out of that into a world full of noise—television, radio, engines, etc.—and bright lights, colors, and constant advertisement is jarring to say the least. This rapid transition is probably the most pronounced and anxiety-inducing for me. However, it is also the thing that seems to balance out the fastest.

While the world you return to may feel foreign, the adaptation period is often shorter than the depression stage and can lead to some truly helpful changes. More exercise, less stuff, a reduction in noise and visual stimulation, and perhaps, a newfound appreciation and incorporation of time in nature into your daily life.

Alienation from Family and Friends

As you can see, there will likely be a lot going on mentally after you get done walking, and in times of mental stress, having a support network is crucial. Unfortunately, it can be difficult for family and friends who have not had similar experiences to be able to understand what is going on for you. They may even struggle to understand the changes you went through on trail. The six months or so that you spent walking felt like six months to them . . . but perhaps a

Heather Tip

As we mentioned in chapter 6, metabolism increases temporarily post-exercise. This effect will compound throughout your trip, driving your metabolic consumption higher and higher. As a result, in much the same manner, it will lower gradually once exercise stops. It can take weeks to return to where it was prior to the hike, and if a maintenance exercise schedule is adopted, it might take even longer (or never go all the way back down). It's important to understand that your body is not a car. It doesn't stop consuming fuel when you turn off the exercise. Instead, you'll need to feed it according to the diminishing metabolic rate with the right kinds of foods to aid in recovery from a taxing physical endeavor (see chapter 6 for more on nutrition).

lifetime to you. For them, you stepped out and back into their world in a fairly short period of time; for you, however, you stepped out of your life and into a completely new one in that same time frame. The juxtaposition is often profound.

As you struggle to synthesize your experience and cope with the shock of how loud everything is and how much stuff you own, your family and friends may greet you with simple questions like, "Did you have fun?" But there is no way to sum up your hike in a simple answer.

In the same way, you can't bring others into your perspective and experience. I once shared a hiking movie made by a friend about her CDT hike with my best friends who had never hiked. Their attention span was limited to about thirty minutes. Meanwhile I was riveted and emotional. I connected with the experience. They simply saw a woman walking through pretty scenery and talking about drinking cow-poo water.

To cope with this unmooring, I have found that staying in touch with people from the trail is key. I have a wide network of friends in the hiking community, many of whom I've never hiked with. Yet we understand the stories, the emotions, the grief, and the joy of the trail in a way no one else can. Connecting with hiking friends, especially in the weeks immediately after completing a hike, can be a godsend for coping with the feeling of alienation from those you were previously close to.

It's important to not judge those who don't understand for their inability to do so. And though you may find that some of the people from your pre-trail life will not be ones that you choose to have in your life after the trail (or vice versa), this outcome is not inevitable.

Returning home to a relationship with a romantic partner may require special care, both before your trip and when you return. Your return as a potentially different person, and one who is coping with major mental adaptations after a long hike, can put a huge strain on a partnership. Several of my relationships have ended, at least in part, as a result of my time on trail. You may find that counseling helps to facilitate discussions around the changes. Your partner may also find that talking to another long-distance hiker or a hiker's partner may help with perspective. The most important thing is to keep the lines of communication open before, during, and after the hike.

COMMON PHYSICAL CHALLENGES OF REINTEGRATION

Though many hikers spend time physically preparing for a long hike, few consider what happens to their bodies afterward. Hikers vary in how much they physically push themselves, and every body responds differently to the demands of a long hike, yet there are two categories of physical challenges that commonly arise for most hikers: post-trail weight gain and HPA axis dysfunction. For some, these changes are expected; for others, they're a surprise. Learning about them before your trip allows you to make decisions during your hike that can mitigate their effects. After experiencing adrenal exhaustion after my PCT hike, and the months required to

return to baseline, I (Katie) now understand how to reduce the likelihood of it happening again.

This section covers the two most common post-trail physical challenges, and the next section offers strategies to mitigate both the mental and physical challenges of reintegration.

Post-Trail Weight Gain

One common physical change long-distance hikers experience on trail is weight loss: most hikers lose at least some weight (and in many cases a lot), and the longer the hike, the more likely this is to occur. As a hiker's appetite

Heather Tip

As an ultrarunner, I always felt a certain pressure to start running again right after a race. More than once I hobbled my way through a run the day after completing a 100-mile race. While getting blood flow circulating after something intense is important, a 1-mile walk would have been more beneficial! I see many hikers fall into the same mental trap for various reasons. ● *Like Katie, I've dealt with HPA axis dysfunction after long endeavors because I didn't allow for enough rest. In recent years I've learned to move in different ways and only when I want to. For me, yoga is the ideal activity to engage in after a long hike. It satisfies the urge to stay active while remaining low impact enough to promote healing rather than further depletion. The mental benefits are a great bonus to the post-hike state as well. Other activities could include low-impact/low-intensity exercises such as swimming, cycling, and walking (e.g., around the neighborhood).* ● *It's inevitable that you'll lose the fitness that you had on trail. But our bodies are not meant to perform at that level forever. All successful elite athletes use mesocycles of training, alternating higher output periods with recovery periods, akin to the strategies outlined in chapter 7. The period after your hike is a recovery mesocycle. While you will lose the fitness you had on trail, proper recovery means you can work your way back to that level more easily in the future.*

ramps up over the course of a trip, many fear the post-trail weight gain that may occur when they are no longer hiking from dawn to dusk. Each body reacts differently to an extended backpacking trip though, so for some hikers, post-trail weight gain may be necessary to get back to a healthy baseline. For others, the weight loss is welcome and they hope to maintain their new physique afterward.

After your hike, the fact that you are no longer exercising for ten or more hours per day obviously plays a role in post-trail weight gain, but there are additional factors at play as well. The first, as any thru-hiker will tell you, is that your hiker hunger does not disappear overnight. During the course of a long hike, your body becomes accustomed to eating enough to meet a high level of exertion, and it takes time for your brain to recalibrate to a new, lower level of daily activity. Appetite gradually balances back out to match your energy output, but it takes a few weeks. During that window, be patient with yourself and focus on nourishing your body with the strategies covered in this section.

In addition to the changing calorie-balance equation, brain chemistry changes may also play a role in post-trail weight gain. Exercise is known to increase levels of the feel-good neurotransmitter dopamine. On a long backpacking trip, your body is conditioned to expect hours of daily exercise, keeping dopamine high. The abrupt reduction in exercise may result in lower levels of dopamine, which are known to stimulate hunger. Stress may also be a contributor: As discussed in chapter 5, mental and emotional stress increase cortisol production, and chronically high cortisol increases cravings for sugar and fat, which can contribute to weight gain. For this reason, supporting your mental and emotional health is just as important to maintaining your post-trail physique as paying attention to diet and exercise.

HPA Axis Dysregulation

Despite your undoubtedly fantastic levels of physical fitness and endurance when you finish a long hike, it's important to recognize that your body is almost certainly in a depleted state. The level of depletion can be mitigated by preparing yourself for resilient health through the strategies outlined in chapter 5 as well as by fueling yourself well on trail with the strategies from chapter 6, but still, a long hike is demanding on the body.

Recall from chapter 5 that chronic stress in any form, including overtraining, can cause dysregulation of the HPA axis, the body's stress-response system. This is commonly referred to as "adrenal fatigue," the lay term for a disruption in the function of the HPA axis. HPA axis dysregulation exists on a spectrum, so it's possible to have very mild symptoms or to have full-blown adrenal exhaustion. It's important to be aware of symptoms and catch them early because the longer you overstress your body, the longer it takes to fully recover.

It's not uncommon for thru-hikers to want to take advantage of their newfound fitness after their hike by planning to participate in running

Heather Tip

It can be hard to launch right back into life while feeling fatigued after a long hike and even harder to fight the urge to start training again. The solution often comes in a caffeinated beverage. However, I strongly recommend against caffeine in the first few weeks after a long hike. This includes coffee, tea, energy drinks, supplements, and soda. ● "But I'm so tired all the time!" ● Good. Take a nap. ● When you aren't covering up your body's signals, you might be surprised at how clearly it tells you that it really just wants rest. The more you listen and give it what it's craving, the faster you'll recoup the losses from accumulated fatigue and reach that point where you're ready to move from recovery to the next stage.

events like marathons. I did this as well. This can be troublesome for a couple of reasons: The first is that backpacking and running use different mechanics, and therefore good backpacking fitness doesn't equate to high performance in running. A more overlooked factor is that your body is overstressed and undernourished at the end of a thru-hike and may not be in as ideal a condition to compete as you expect.

While I was on the PCT, I submitted my application for an 18-mile trail race in Asheville, North Carolina, where I lived at the time. Admission to this popular race was by lottery only and I'd applied multiple times previously without luck. During my last month on the PCT, I got the email that I was in—I was thrilled! According to my plan, I would allow myself one week of rest after the PCT and still have two months to train. The first part of the plan—the rest week—went great. Then once training was set to begin, I hit a wall. I couldn't run more than a few miles without extreme fatigue. My legs felt like 100-pound weights. I gave myself another week of rest and tried again. My body simply refused, and I had to make the heart-wrenching decision to give up my spot in the race. I eventually found out I had overstressed my body and had adrenal dysfunction. It wasn't just hiking the PCT that set the stage for my health challenges afterward, though—a combination of pre-existing factors and emotional distress caused my "stress cup" to overflow at that time.

Of course, most hikers' post-trail experiences aren't as extreme as mine was. However, I do know many hikers who undergo extreme post-trail fatigue that lasts for weeks. This is why pre-trail adrenal health is covered in chapter 5 and in the Adventure Ready online course. Post-trail strategies to recover more quickly are presented here.

Keep in mind that you don't need to wait until you finish your hike to set yourself up for faster recovery and an easier reintegration period. The

Heather Tip

I used to crave cheeseburgers, milkshakes, and fries loaded with ketchup after hiking. It was a clockwork craving for many years, even after only a few days in the backcountry. However, I noticed something interesting: as my foods changed on trail (and off), so did my cravings. These days the first thing I want post hike is a bottle of kombucha and a mega salad—one seed and one feed. As I learned to nourish my body on trail, my body also began to communicate different needs. While I may still sometimes want a burger, my body generally gets the nutrition it needs on trail, so it focuses its requests on maintaining my gut biome balance in towns and after a hike.

best way to ease the post-trail transition is to go in with the most resilient health possible and to take care of yourself on trail (see chapter 5). You can reduce the amount of lean muscle mass lost during your hike by consuming adequate protein. More lean muscle helps mitigate post-trail weight gain because muscle is more metabolically active than fat and therefore will burn more calories even while you're at rest.

Furthermore, you can minimize post-trail weight gain by not becoming addicted to nutrient-poor, processed food on your hike. Your taste buds change in response to the food that you eat, and food scientists are well paid to create combinations of fat, salt, and sugar to keep you coming back for more. I've met more than a few hikers who have struggled to readjust their diets after months of consuming highly processed foods on trail. Prioritizing whole foods and consuming blood-sugar–balanced meals during your hike, as discussed in chapter 6, will not only support steady energy but will further support adrenal health during your post-hike transition.

STRATEGIES FOR REINTEGRATION

Now that you know what to expect, the next best way to prepare yourself for reintegration is to have a toolbox of strategies you can use as needed to navigate the transition. Use the strategies outlined here to benefit your physical, mental, and emotional well-being so that you can transition into post-trail life with more ease and recover more quickly for your next adventure.

Before you engage in any of the following practices, bear in mind that the number-one way to support yourself after a big adventure is to listen to your body and honor its needs. Your body and mind need time to relax and repair after you have demanded so much of it. The longer, harder, and more intense the hike, the more important it is to be intentional about a recovery period, even if your ego is trying to convince you otherwise.

Once you have set yourself up for a smoother transition into post-trail life by taking care of your physical health, you can further boost your mental health with additional strategies that allow you to feel safe, grounded, and supported. These include planning for life after the trail, creating routine, seeking counseling, and staying connected with the trail community.

Movement

The science-backed benefits of movement are many, including cardiovascular health, better energy, deeper sleep, improved mood, healthy immune function, and more. In the context of reintegration, we recommend a regular movement practice primarily for the mental health benefits. It's important to allow yourself time to rest and repair after a hike, but maintaining a practice of light activity can be helpful.

There is no one right amount or form of exercise for everyone. Gauge the right level of intensity for yourself by listening to your body. A guideline to keep in mind is that exercise should energize you rather than drain you. If you're finding yourself exhausted after workouts, it may be your body's signal to ease up for now. Another key indicator is your level of motivation.

Your mind needs a break from forcing yourself to do hard things just as much as your body does. This is especially true if you pushed your physical, mental, and emotional limits on your hike. If you're forcing yourself through your workouts day after day, your mind and body are telling you to rest.

After every thru-hike, I am tempted to jump back into training before my body is truly ready. My type-A mind convinces me that I have had enough rest and that I should start training again to take advantage of my fitness level. I end up creating an overly ambitious training schedule, sticking to it for a week or two until either my body or mind rebels, and then getting down on myself for not following through. When I was in this phase after my CDT hike, Heather said something to me that struck a chord. She reminded me that nature operates in seasons and so do we; there are seasons of activity and seasons of rest. We need downtime in order to prepare for times of maximal output.

To get a more objective measurement on your body's readiness for exercise, consider a heart rate variability (HRV) monitor. HRV measures the variation in time between each heartbeat. It provides a snapshot into how well your body is balancing the parasympathetic and sympathetic branches of your autonomic nervous system. A lower HRV indicates that your body is under more stress, needs recovery time, and is therefore not in a good state for intense exercise.

Lab Testing

Another way to get an objective assessment on your health is to do lab testing. Having lab work done allows you to "take a look under the hood" so that you can get an objective measurement of metrics that aren't easily assessed from the outside. These tests provide insight into your body's level of stress and inflammation and your overall nutritional status, including any deficiencies. A few tests you may wish to request include:

- Micronutrient testing to inform you of any deficiencies
- High-sensitivity C-reactive protein (hs-CRP), which can indicate levels of inflammation in the body
- Complete blood count (CBC) to evaluate your overall health and potentially detect any infections

Results from lab tests can inform your post-trail dietary and/or supplementation strategy.

Nourishing Your Body

Food provides us with the calories, micronutrients, and macronutrients we need for energy, but it's so much more. It has the ability to create health or destroy it. It informs gene expression. It helps our bodies repair and impacts levels of inflammation. Food affects mood, mental clarity, immune function, and the release of various hormones, both the timing and volume. It can also help you maintain healthy body weight and restore adrenal health after a long-distance hike. Food is a powerful source of healing!

Chapter 6 outlined the importance of nourishing your body with nutrient-dense whole foods. If you relied solely on processed foods on your hike and you're having a hard time kicking the habit when you return home, focusing on whole foods will ease the transition. The water, fiber, and nutrients increase satiation, helping you to keep calorie intake in check while your hiker hunger normalizes. Fiber also helps with microbiome support and clearing excess hormones. Be sure to eat enough protein for your body and level of activity and consume healthy fat at each meal to nourish hormones and increase satiation. Refer back to chapter 6 for a detailed discussion of balancing macronutrients to stabilize blood sugar and energy levels.

A word of caution: you may be tempted to force yourself to undereat to try to maintain your trail physique; however, this usually results in a rebound binge. I've also heard of hikers who

decide to do a juice "cleanse" to "detox" as a way to repent after months of eating junk on trail. For some this can be a needed psychological reset with food, but for many it backfires. Your body has built-in detoxification systems and you naturally "detox" every day via your liver, kidneys, and colon. You can support this process by eating nutrient-dense foods, drinking plenty of water, and eliminating substances that burden the liver, such as caffeine, alcohol, and sugar.

Microbiome Support

As discussed in chapter 5, your gut health directly impacts the health of nearly every aspect of well-being, including your energy, immunity, mood, and digestion. Furthermore, important hormones and neurotransmitters, including 90 percent of serotonin, are produced in the digestive tract. Moderately high levels of serotonin are associated with positive mood and feelings of calm and mental alertness.

Taking care of your microbiome is one of the best ways you can support your physical, mental, and emotional health after your hike. Due to a lack of fresh foods and sources of probiotics on trail as well as an abundance of microbiome-harming foods, most hikers benefit from focusing extra attention on gut repair during reintegration. This can be done by including more soluble fiber in the diet, increasing intake of probiotic foods and supplements, and minimizing foods and substances that destroy the microbiome. Refer to the seed-and-feed strategy in chapter 5 for more details on optimizing gut health.

Sunlight

As diurnal creatures, sunlight is one of the most powerful regulators of our internal clock, which plays an important role in overall health. The body's internal clock governs our natural cycles (circadian rhythms) including sleep and wakefulness, as well as hunger, mental alertness, mood,

REINTEGRATION STRATEGIES	
HEALTH STRATEGIES	**ADDITIONAL STRATEGIES**
Sunlight	Have a plan
Movement	Create routine
Microbiome support	Seek counseling
Eat to nourish your body	Connect with the trail community

stress, heart function, and immunity. Researchers have found connections between disrupted circadian rhythms and traffic accidents, workplace injuries, and chronic health issues, ranging from diabetes to heart disease and cognitive decline. The time-keeping region of the brain, the suprachiasmatic nucleus (SCN), is located above the point where the optic nerve fibers cross. This enables the SCN to keep time based on cues from light in the environment.

The internal clock impacts the secretion and rhythms of serotonin, melatonin, and cortisol. Exposure to bright light in the morning resets our cortisol rhythm, which peaks a few hours after sunrise and gradually falls throughout the day. It also sets the clock for melatonin production to increase fourteen to sixteen hours later, allowing you to enter into sleep more easily. This melatonin-phase advancement can be effective against insomnia and seasonal affective disorder as well. Many hikers who end their hikes in autumn fall prey to both conditions. Exposure to sunlight also increases the brain's production of serotonin, the precursor to melatonin.

This daily sunlight exposure, especially at certain times of day, is probably even more important than we realize. Exposure to the natural cycles of daylight (and reduced exposure to artificial light at night) may be one of the many reasons we feel so good on a thru-hike. To set your clock once you're back home, get as much bright light as you can before noon. Particularly, aim to get natural light—even just

ten minutes—within the first hour after waking. Being outside is the most effective option as daylight is fifty to one hundred times stronger than indoor light. For precise measurements, test different indoor and outdoor environments with a free app such as Lux Light Meter. Allowing your eyes to take in low-angle, natural light as the sun is setting also supports normal sleep-wake cycles.

In addition to the ability of natural-light exposure to set your internal clock, sunlight also plays an important role in assisting the body with the production of vitamin D. Vitamin D, which is actually a hormone, strengthens bones and muscles, supports the immune system, fights inflammation, boosts mood, and reduces the risk of certain cancers. It's critical for good health!

Most public health campaigns warn against the exposure of too much sun exposure, and while there are certainly dangers to overexposure, sunlight is essential to health. Aim to get daily exposure without getting sunburned. Bonus if your daily sunlight exposure includes time in nature. We already discussed, and you no doubt intuitively know, the myriad physical and mental health benefits of nature immersion.

Planning for Post-Trail Life

Hikers often say "the trail provides." This saying, used to relieve undue concerns, can prevent you from ruminating on things that are outside of your control, but I have witnessed far too many hikers, myself included, attempt to carry this happy-go-lucky outlook into their post-trail lives, hoping that everything (home, income, career path, etc.) will magically fall into place. Even after spending months planning all the details for a big adventure, many people fail to take into account what happens *after* the adventure is over. Having no plan for how you will take care of yourself physically, mentally, and emotionally results in a sense of instability and feeling ungrounded and can compound the challenges you experience during reentry. Taking the time to create a plan for what you will do after the trail is one of the best ways to take care of your future self and set yourself up for an easier transition into post-trail life.

Avoid unnecessary additional stress during reintegration by setting yourself up for greater stability upon your return. Arrange for a stable housing situation (couch-surfing doesn't count), have an income stream lined up and emergency funds that will allow you to relax for a week or two before you need to return to work. Having these foundations covered can do wonders for your mental health. It allows the reintegration period to feel like simply another transition phase you're capable of handling rather than an uphill battle rebuilding your life.

Creating Routine

After my CDT hike, I (Katie) struggled with reintegration despite having a safe home, a steady source of income, and plenty of safety cash in the bank. I was returning to a town I loved, friends that I missed, and the snuggles of my beloved feline fur child. I had achieved my goal and set myself up for post-trail success, yet still I struggled. Everything seemed meaningless, and I felt lost and listless. It was during this time that I discovered how valuable routine can be in creating a sense of safety and stability. I began a morning routine of matcha, yoga, and journaling, which provided a sense of optimism and added meaning to my day. I implemented

consistent sleep and wake times and felt my sense of well-being improve. My days began to have structure and purpose. Routines can provide a foundation while you get your footing and explore next steps during reentry. They can be built around any practices that are meaningful to you, such as meditation, yoga, art, music, etc. Follow the golden thread of what inspires you.

Counseling

During times of great transition, assembling a dedicated support system can be indispensable to your well-being. A thru-hike is a life-changing event for many people. Values and priorities change. Perhaps you set out on a long-distance hike to find clarity and you return feeling more confused than before. A therapist or counselor can help you process the experience, support you through challenging emotions, and guide you with rediscovering your purpose and zest for life. Many counseling options exist, from in-person talk therapy to online options such as Talkspace and BetterHelp (see Additional Resources).

Connecting with the Trail Community

No one will understand what you've just gone through and what you're currently going through as much as a fellow hiker. Both Heather and I have found that staying connected with trail friends reduces the sense of alienation you feel upon returning home and allows you to support one another during reintegration.

Another great way to stay involved in the trail community is to join trail organizations. Trail organizations always need volunteers. Whether you want to do trail maintenance, organize local trail cleanups, or share your hard-earned knowledge with up-and-coming hikers, there are myriad ways to get involved and give back to the trail community from which you gained so much. Joining trail crews and volunteering my time on the board of the American Long-Distance

Hiking Association-West and in other capacities has added so much richness to my life over the years. I've made lifelong friends, become part of a supportive trail community, and found a meaningful way to share my love of the outdoors by teaching those who are new to backpacking.

Connecting to the trail community after your hike also benefits you when it's time for your next adventure. The trail community is full of knowledgeable individuals who love to share their experiences and who understand your deep call to adventure. Combining the self-efficacy and confidence you've gained from your experience on the trail with a supportive community helps you to create the life you desire—and to be ready for your next long-distance hike.

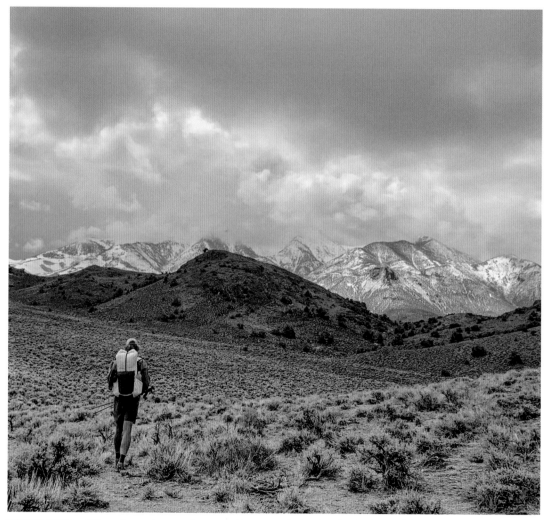

With knowledge, skills, and experience under your belt, your next adventure is simply a decision away.

WORKSHEETS & CHECKLISTS

ITINERARY & EMERGENCY CONTACT WORKSHEET

It is important to leave an itinerary and list of emergency contacts with a trusted person for every trip you take. Be sure to include the full names of everyone in your party and their emergency contacts as well.

ROUTE NAME & BRIEF DESCRIPTION
(include name of land area, e.g., North Cascades National Park, as well as the closest city and state):

DATE TRIP BEGINS		DATE TRIP ENDS	
PROJECTED # OF NIGHTS IN THE BACKCOUNTRY		DATE CONSIDERED OVERDUE *(when to contact authorities)*	
ORIGINATING TRAILHEAD		TERMINATING TRAILHEAD	
RETURNING TO THE SAME TRAILHEAD?	Y N		
VEHICLE(S) LEFT AT ORIGINATING TRAILHEAD?	Y N	VEHICLE(S) LEFT AT TERMINATING TRAILHEAD?	Y N
VEHICLE(S) MAKE/MODEL/COLOR/YEAR	**PLATE** *(including state)*	VEHICLE(S) MAKE/MODEL/COLOR/YEAR	**PLATE** *(including state)*

DESCRIPTION OF GEAR

BACKPACK BRAND/COLOR/SIZE	
TENT BRAND/COLOR/STYLE	
OUTER LAYERS *(e.g., red rain jacket, blue puffy)*	
SHOE BRAND/MODEL/SIZE	
OTHER PERTINENT GEAR DESCRIPTORS	

ITINERARY & EMERGENCY CONTACT WORKSHEET (CONT.)

PHYSICAL DESCRIPTION FOR ALL MEMBERS OF THE PARTY
(include images of your backpack, tent & yourself/others in party for maximum usefulness)

NAME	AGE	HEIGHT	WEIGHT	GENDER	HAIR COLOR	EYE COLOR	SKIN COLOR

PROJECTED ITINERARY

NIGHT	CAMPSITE	*(use names of primitive sites/shelters/GPS coordinates/geographic descriptors, not just mileages from start, although those are important too)*
1		
2		
3		
4		
5		
6		
7		
8		
9		
10		
11		
12		
13		
14		

ITINERARY & EMERGENCY CONTACT WORKSHEET (CONT.)

EMERGENCY NUMBERS

LAND MANAGEMENT AGENCY	
EMERGENCY PHONE NUMBER	
LOCAL EMERGENCY PROVIDER	
PHONE NUMBER	

ADDITIONAL PHONE NUMBERS & EMERGENCY CONTACTS
(include emergency contact information for each member of the party)

ASSESSING RISK CHECKLIST

**ROUTE NAME &
BRIEF DESCRIPTION**

WEATHER RISKS

TIME OF YEAR TRIP IS PLANNED

*Typical weather for the area during that
time (hot, cold, dry, wet, average temps, etc.)*

**LIST ACTIONABLE LEARNING NEEDED
BEFORE ATTEMPTING TRIP**

*(climate research, weather forecast, how
to diagnose and treat heat illness, etc.)*

**MITIGATION GEAR & CLOTHING
NEEDED FOR YOUR ROUTE
BASED ON THE ABOVE**

ROUTE PREPAREDNESS & NAVIGATIONAL RISKS

Refer to chapter 4 for more information.

HOW IS MY ROUTE MARKED?	
DO I HAVE TOPOGRAPHICAL MAPS FOR ITS ENTIRETY?	
HAVE I HIKED IT BEFORE? DO I HAVE SUPPLEMENTAL NAVIGATIONAL DATA? *(GPS, Farout app, etc.)* **WHAT ELSE MIGHT I NEED?**	
DO I HAVE EVERYTHING FROM THE NAVIGATION & ROUTE PREPAREDNESS CHECKLIST? *(See following checklists.)* **WHAT ADDITIONAL ITEMS DO I NEED?**	
DO I HAVE A COMPLETE BETA PACKET? *(See following checklists.)* **WHAT, IF ANYTHING, IS MISSING?**	

NAVIGATION & ROUTE PREPAREDNESS CHECKLIST

☐ TOPOGRAPHIC MAPS FOR THE ROUTE AND SURROUNDING AREA

☐ MAGNETIC COMPASS WITH MANUALLY ADJUSTABLE DECLINATION

☐ GPS UNIT OR PHONE APP WITH BACKGROUND MAPS AND TRACKLOG OF THE ROUTE *(optional)*

☐ BETA PACKET *(see next checklist and chapter 4)*

☐ WATERPROOFING FOR NAVIGATIONAL SUPPLIES

☐ WATER SOURCE LIST

☐ ALTERNATE ROUTE DESCRIPTIONS *(and marked on topographic maps)*

☐ PLB *(personal locator beacon)*

BETA PACKET CHECKLIST

☐ TOPOGRAPHIC MAPS MARKED WITH ALTERNATE ROUTES

☐ PHOTOS OF LANDMARKS *(especially important for cross-country travel)*

☐ ROUTE DESCRIPTION*(s)*

WHO WILL I BE HIKING WITH? _____

WHO IS MY EMERGENCY CONTACT? _____

☐ HAVE I PROVIDED THEM AN ITINERARY & EMERGENCY CONTACT WORKSHEET WITH THE NECESSARY INFORMATION TO RELAY TO EMERGENCY PERSONNEL IF I AM DELAYED?

PHYSICAL PREPAREDNESS & INJURY RISKS

Refer to chapter 7 for more information.

AM I CERTAIN THAT I AM PHYSICALLY CAPABLE OF COMPLETING THE ROUTE IN THE TIME FRAME I'VE GIVEN MYSELF?

IF NOT, WHAT DO I STILL NEED TO DO TO BE PREPARED?

WHAT INJURIES ARE LIKELY TO OCCUR ON THIS ROUTE?

WHAT WILL I NEED TO TREAT OR MITIGATE THE ABOVE?

DO I, OR A MEMBER OF THE PARTY, HAVE BASIC WILDERNESS FIRST-AID TRAINING AND THE SUPPLIES TO TREAT INJURY?

WHAT ADDITIONAL SKILLS MIGHT BE NEEDED, AND HOW DO I ACQUIRE THEM?

ANIMAL & HUMAN INTERACTION RISKS

LIST THE ANIMALS MOST LIKELY TO BE ENCOUNTERED AND THAT MAY POSE RISKS ON THIS TRIP
(research each animal and learn about their habits and what to do if encountered; see Additional Resources for more information)

AM I LIKELY TO ENCOUNTER OTHER PEOPLE ON THIS TRIP?	
WHAT HUMAN INTERACTIONS ARE POSSIBLE THAT MAY INVOLVE RISK?	
HOW CAN I PREVENT THESE SCENARIOS FROM OCCURRING?	
WHAT WILL I DO IF I ENCOUNTER SOMEONE WHOM I DON'T TRUST OR WHO IS ACTING VIOLENTLY/ERRATICALLY?	

POTENTIAL WATER & SNOW RISKS

WHICH FORM OF WATER TREATMENT DO I NEED?	
SWEAT RATE IN SIMILAR CONDITIONS *(see Additional Resources)*	
AMOUNT OF WATER-CARRYING CAPACITY NEEDED	
LIST OF ALTERNATE ROUTES IN CASE OF WATER OR SNOW HAZARDS *(be certain to include them in the research and beta creation phase)*	

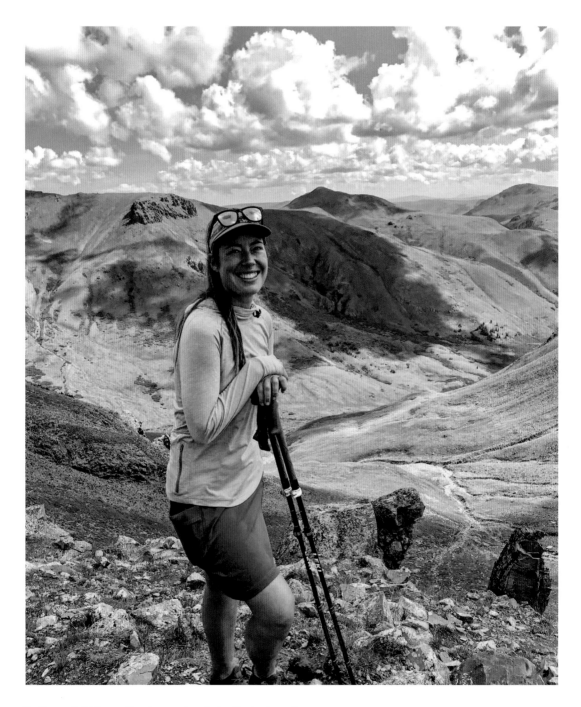

Feeling grateful for another day spent exploring the backcountry

ADDITIONAL RESOURCES

Here is a curated list of resources you may find useful in your planning. For additional information as well as assignments and supplements for each topic, check out our Adventure Ready online course and Backpacker Academy courses at https://katiegerber.teachable.com/courses.

CHAPTER 1: PLANNING YOUR BACKPACKING TRIP: AN OVERVIEW

American Long-Distance Hiking Association–West Rucks: www.aldhawest.org/rucks

Backpacker Long Trails: Mastering the Art of the Thru-Hike by Liz Thomas

Craig's PCT Planner: https://pctplanner.com

Leave No Trace Principles: https://lnt.org

National Oceanic and Atmospheric Administration (NOAA): www.weather.gov

CHAPTER 2: GEAR SELECTION

Leave No Trace: https://lnt.org

Trail Tested: A Thru-Hiker's Guide to Ultralight Hiking and Backpacking by Justin Lichter

The Ultimate Hiker's Gear Guide by Andrew Skurka

Cottage Industry Gear

Branwyn (women's wool blend innerwear): https://branwyn.com

Enlightened Equipment (backpacking quilts, apparel): https://enlightenedequipment.com

Gossamer Gear (packs, shelters, trekking poles, accessories): www.gossamergear.com

Hyperlite Mountain Gear (packs, shelters): www.hyperlitemountaingear.com

Katabatic Gear (backpacking quilts): https://katabaticgear.com

Mountain Laurel Designs (shelters, packs): https://mountainlaureldesigns.com

Six Moon Designs (backpacks, tents, and umbrellas): www.sixmoondesigns.com

Tarptent (tents): www.tarptent.com

Ultralight Adventure Equipment (packs): www.ula-equipment.com

YAMA Mountain Gear (tents and tarps): https://yamamountaingear.com

Zpacks (shelters, packs): https://zpacks.com

Mainstream Gear

Leki (trekking poles): www.leki.com/us

Montbell (outerwear, technical apparel, sleeping bags, wide variety of backpacking gear): www.montbell.us

REI (outdoor-gear retail cooperative with a generous return policy): www.rei.com

Sawyer Products (water filters, bug repellents, sunscreen): https://sawyer.com

Second-Hand Gear

Patagonia Worn Wear: https://wornwear.patagonia.com

REI Good & Used: www.rei.com/used

Discounted Gear

Backcountry: www.backcountry.com

The Clymb: www.theclymb.com

REI Outlet: www.rei.com/rei-garage

Steep and Cheap: www.steepandcheap.com

Review Websites

Backpacking Light: https://backpackinglight.com

Gear Junkie: https://gearjunkie.com

Gear Lab: www.outdoorgearlab.com

Treeline Review: www.treelinereview.com (our top pick)

CHAPTER 3: BACKCOUNTRY SAFETY

Backpacker Academy: Stay Safe in the Backcountry online course: https://katiegerber.teachable.com/p/backpacker-academy-backcountry-safety

Animal Research Resources

Bears: www.bearsmart.com/play/bear-encounters

Florida snakes: https://floridahikes.com/venomous-snakes

Mountain lions: www.fs.usda.gov/visit/know-before-you-go/mountain-lions, https://mountainlion.org

Rattlesnakes: www.wta.org/news/signpost/how-to-hike-in-rattlesnake-country

Ticks: www.cdc.gov/niosh/topics/tick-borne/resources.html

Venomous snakes: www.cdc.gov/niosh/topics/snakes/default.html

Wolves: http://bcparks.ca/explore/misc/wolves

Snow and Water

Snow Safety: www.backpacker.com/skills/how-to-cross-a-spring-snowfield

Sweat Rate Calculator: www.cdc.gov/nceh/hsb/extreme/Heat_Illness/Sweat%20Rate%20Calculation.pdf

Water-Crossing Safety: www.pcta.org/discover-the-trail/backcountry-basics/water/stream-crossing-safety

CHAPTER 4: NAVIGATION & ROUTE PREPAREDNESS

Backpacker Academy: Become a Better Backcountry Navigator online course: https://katiegerber.teachable.com/p/backpacker-academy-backcountry-navigation

CalTopo: https://caltopo.com

Declination Resources from NOAA: www.ngdc.noaa.gov/geomag/declination.shtml

Farout: https://faroutguides.com

Gaia GPS: www.gaiagps.com

CHAPTER 5: CREATING A RESILIENT BODY

Adventure Ready online course: https://katiegerber.teachable.com/p/adventure-ready

Environmental Working Group: www.ewg.org

The Huberman Lab Podcast (on neuroscience and how the brain impacts our body, behaviors, and overall health): https://hubermanlab.libsyn.com

Independent Research on Supplements: https://examine.com

The Inflammation Spectrum by Dr. Will Cole

Mindfulness, Meditation, and Sleep Apps

www.calm.com

www.headspace.com

www.oakmeditation.com

CHAPTER 6: PERFORMANCE NUTRITION & BACKCOUNTRY MEAL PLANNING

BMR Calculator: https://exrx.net/Calculators/CalRequire

Metabolic Efficiency Training by Bob Seebohar

Peak Nutrition: Smart Fuel for Outdoor Adventure by Maria Hines and Mercedes Pollmeier

Food Tracking Apps

https://cronometer.com

www.myfitnesspal.com

Backcountry Meal Planning Resources

Healthy Hiker Grocery Guide; Eat for Endurance eBook; Healthy Lightweight Eating for Hikers 101 (online course): http://katiegerber.com/freebies

Sample smoothie recipe: http://katiegerber.com/skip-the-sugar-crash-trail-smoothie

Additional healthy backpacking recipes: www.eathikelove.com/recipes

Tips for estimating stove-fuel needs

www.msrgear.com/blog/stoves-101-how-much
-fuel-should-i-carry

www.rei.com/learn/expert-advice/how-much
-stove-fuel-should-i-take-on-my-backpacking
-trip.html

CHAPTER 7: PHYSICAL PREPARATION

American Council on Exercise (ACE) Fit Exercise
Library: www.acefitness.org/education-and
-resources/lifestyle/exercise-library

Eco-conscious Self-Care Products for Home and
the Trail: www.rawlogy.com

*ROAR: How to Match Your Food and Fitness to
Your Unique Female Physiology for Optimum
Performance, Great Health, and a Strong, Lean
Body for Life* by Selene Yeager and Stacy T. Sims

CHAPTER 8: MENTAL & EMOTIONAL PREPARATION

*Endure: Mind, Body, and the Curiously Elastic Limits
of Human Performance* by Alex Hutchinson

Information on Meditation and Mindfulness (see chapter 5 for meditation apps)

www.mayoclinic.org/tests-procedures/meditation
/in-depth/meditation/art-20045858

www.mindful.org/meditation/mindfulness-getting
-started

Mental Preparation for the AT: *Appalachian Trails: A
Psychological and Emotional Guide to Successfully
Thru-Hiking the Appalachian Trail* by Zach Davis

CHAPTER 9: REINTEGRATION

Counseling Resources

www.betterhelp.com

www.talkspace.com

Thorough discussion of depression:
www.mayoclinic.org/diseases-conditions
/depression/symptoms-causes/syc-20356007

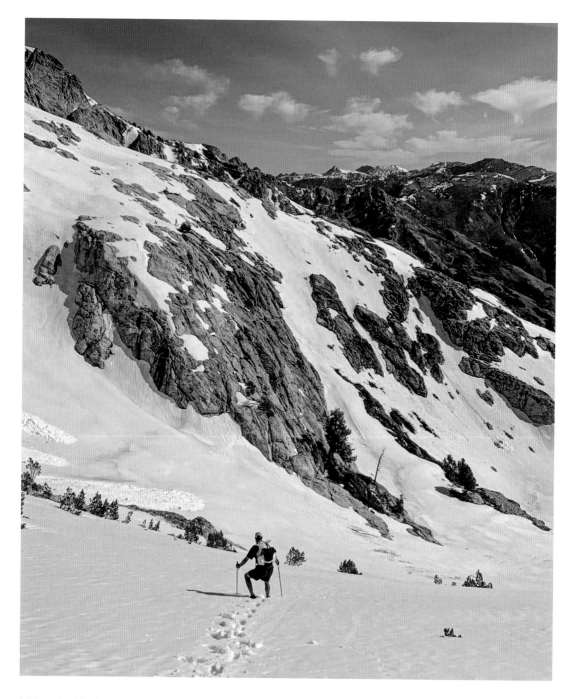

A late spring hike in Nevada's Ruby Mountains provides stunning views and ample opportunity for adventure.

SELECTED SOURCES

This list includes the primary scientific publications and peer-reviewed research that informed the data and advice shared in chapters 5 and 6.

CHAPTER 5: CREATING A RESILIENT BODY

Hewlings, Susan J., and Douglas S. Kalman. "Curcumin: A Review of Its Effects on Human Health." *Foods* 6, no. 10 (Oct 2017): 92, https://doi.org/10.3390/foods6100092.

Panossian, Alexander, and Georg Wikman. "Pharmacology of *Schisandra chinensis* Bail.: An overview of Russian research and uses in medicine." *Journal of Ethnopharmacology* 118, no. 2 (July 2008): 183–212, https://doi.org/10.1016/j.jep.2008.04.020.

Punja, Salima, Larissa Shamseer, Karin Olson, and Sunita Vohra. "*Rhodiola rosea* for mental and physical fatigue in nursing students: A randomized controlled trial." *PLoS One* 9, no. 9 (Sept 2014): https://doi.org/10.1371/journal.pone.0108416.

Sellami, Maha, Olfa Slimeni, Andrzej Pokrywka, et al. "Herbal medicine for sports: A review." *Journal of the International Society of Sports Nutrition* 15, no. 14 (March 2018): https://doi.org/10.1186/s12970-018-0218-y.

Shenoy, Shweta, Udesh Chaskar, Jaspal S. Sandhu, and Madan Mohan Paadhi. "Effects of eight-week supplementation of Ashwagandha on cardiorespiratory endurance in elite Indian cyclists." *Journal of Ayurveda and Integrative Medicine* 3, no. 4 (Dec 2012): 209–14, https://dx.doi.org/10.4103%2F0975-9476.104444.

Tuli, Hardeep S., Sardul S. Sandhu, and A. K. Sharma. "Pharmacological and therapeutic potential of *Cordyceps* with special reference to Cordycepin." *3 Biotech* 4, (Feb 2014): 1–12, https://doi.org/10.1007/s13205-013-0121-9.

White, Mathew P., Ian Alcock, James Grellier, et al. "Spending at least 120 minutes a week in nature is associated with good health and well-being." *Scientific Reports* 9, (June 2019): https://doi.org/10.1038/s41598-019-44097-3.

CHAPTER 6: PERFORMANCE NUTRITION & BACKCOUNTRY MEAL PLANNING

Berardi, John M., Thomas B. Price, Eric E. Noreen, Peter W. Lemon. "Postexercise muscle glycogen recovery enhanced with a carbohydrate-protein supplement." *Medicine and Science in Sports and Exercise* 38, no. 6 (June 2006): 1106-13, https://doi.org/10.1249/01.mss.0000222826.49358.f3.

Burke, L. M., G. R. Collier, S. K. Beasley, et al. "Effect of coingestion of fat and protein with carbohydrate feedings on muscle glycogen storage." *Journal of Applied Physiology (1985)* 78, no. 6 (June 1995): 2187–92, https://doi.org/10.1152/jappl.1995.78.6.2187.

Chen, Xiaojia, Zhang Zhang, Huijie Yang, et al. "Consumption of ultra-processed foods and health outcomes: A systematic review of epidemiological studies." *Nutrition Journal* 19, no. 86 (Aug 2020): https://doi.org/10.1186/s12937-020-00604-1.

Erith, Samuel, Clyde Williams, Emma Stevenson, Siovhan Chamberlain, Pippa Crews, and Ian Rushbury. "The effect of high carbohydrate meals with different glycemic indices on recovery of performance during prolonged intermittent high-intensity shuttle running." *International Journal of Sport Nutrition and Exercise Metabolism* 16, no. 4 (Aug 2006): 393–404, https://doi.org/10.1123/ijsnem.16.4.393.

Fox, Amanda K., Amy E. Kaufman and Jeffrey F. Horowitz. "Adding fat calories to meals after exercise does not alter glucose tolerance." *Journal of Applied Physiology (1985)* 97, no. 1 (July 2004): 11–6, https://doi.org/10.1152/japplphysiol.01398.2003.

Fuhrman, Joel, Barbara Sarter, Dale Glaser, and Steve Acocella. "Changing perceptions of hunger on a high nutrient density diet." *Nutrition Journal* 9, no. 51 (Nov 2010): https://doi.org/10.1186/1475-2891-9-51.

Gonzalez, Javier T., Cas J. Fuchs, James A. Betts, and Luc J. C. van Loon. "Glucose Plus Fructose Ingestion for Post-Exercise Recovery-Greater than the Sum of Its Parts?" *Nutrients* 9, no. 4 (March 2017): 344, https://doi.org/10.3390/nu9040344.

Hall, Kevin. D., Alexis Ayuketah, Robert Brychta, et al. "Ultra-processed diets cause excess calorie intake and weight gain: An inpatient randomized controlled trial of ad libitum food intake." *Cell Metabolism* 30, no. 1 (July 2019): 67–77, https://doi.org/10.1016/j.cmet.2019.05.008.

Ivy, John L., Harold W. Goforth Jr., Bruce M. Damon, Thomas R. McCauley, Edward C. Parsons and Thomas B. Price. "Early postexercise muscle glycogen recovery is enhanced with a carbohydrate-protein supplement." *Journal of Applied Physiology (1985)* 93, no. 4 (Oct 2002): 1337–44, https://doi.org/10.1152/japplphysiol.00394.2002.

Ivy, John L., A. L. Katz, C. L. Cutler, W. M. Sherman, and E. F. Coyle. "Muscle glycogen synthesis after exercise: effect of time of carbohydrate ingestion." *Journal of Applied Physiology (1985)* 64, no. 4 (April 1988): 1480–5, https://doi.org/10.1152/jappl.1988.64.4.1480. PMID: 3132449.

Ivy, John L., Peter T. Res, Robert C. Sprague, and Matthew O. Widzer. "Effect of a carbohydrate-protein supplement on endurance performance during exercise of varying intensity." *International Journal of Sport Nutrition and Exercise Metabolism* 13, no. 3 (Sep 2003): 382–95, https://doi.org/10.1123/ijsnem.13.3.382.

Jentjens, Roy, and Asker Jeukendrup. "Determinants of post-exercise glycogen synthesis during short-term recovery." *Sports Medicine* 33, no. 2 (Oct 2003): 117–44, https://doi.org/10.2165/00007256-200333020-00004.

Metabolic Efficiency Training. "What Is It?" Accessed March 19, 2021. www.metabolicefficiency.org/what-is-it.

Muscella, Antonella, Erika Stefàno, Paola Lunetti, Loredana Capobianco, and Santo Marsigliante. "The regulation of fat metabolism during aerobic exercise." *Biomolecules* 10, no. 12 (Dec 2020): 1699, https://doi.org/10.3390/biom10121699.

Schoenfeld, Brad Jon, and Alan Albert Aragon. "How much protein can the body use in a single meal for muscle-building? Implications for daily protein distribution." *Journal of the International Society of Sports Nutrition* 15, no. 10 (Feb 2018): https://doi.org/10.1186/s12970-018-0215-1.

Stevenson, Emma, Clyde Williams, Gareth McComb, and Christopher Oram. "Improved recovery from prolonged exercise following the consumption of low glycemic index carbohydrate meals." *International Journal of Sport Nutrition and Exercise Metabolism* 15, no. 4 (Aug 2005): 333–49, https://doi.org/10.1123/ijsnem.15.4.333.

St. Pierre, Brian. "Workout Nutrition Explained." Precision Nutrition. www.precisionnutrition.com/workout-nutrition-explained.

Williamson, Eric. "Nutritional implications for ultra-endurance walking and running events." *Extreme Physiology and Medicine* 5, no. 13 (Nov 2016): https://doi.org/10.1186/s13728-016-0054-0.

Zinöcker Marit K., and Inge A. Lindseth. "The Western diet-microbiome-host interaction and its role in metabolic disease." *Nutrients* 10, no. 3 (March 2018): 365, https://doi.org/10.3390/nu10030365.

INDEX